Surgical Recovery

Edited by Selim Sozen

Published in London, United Kingdom

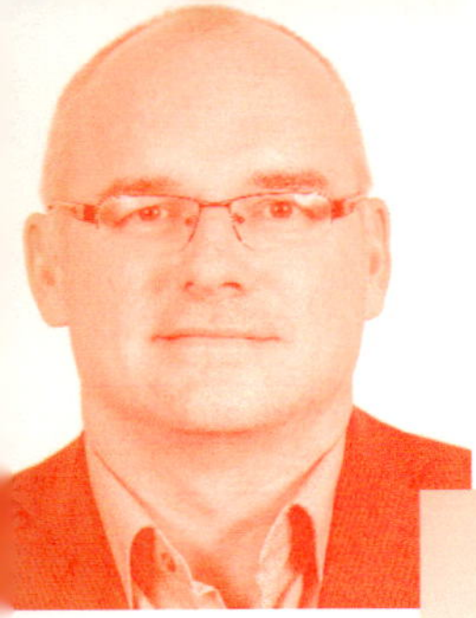
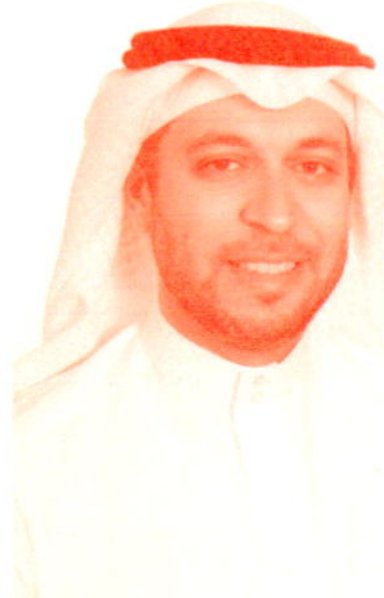
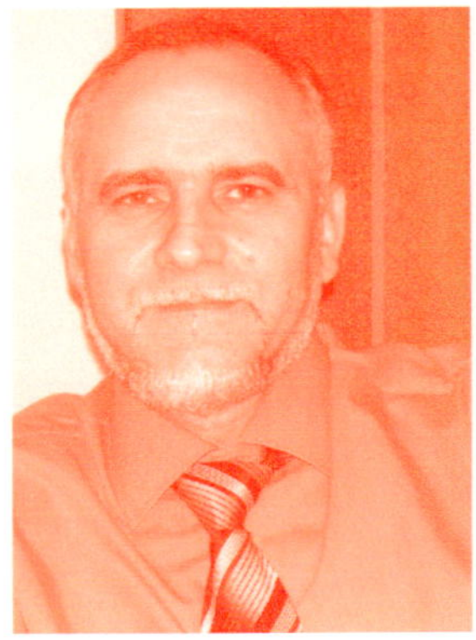
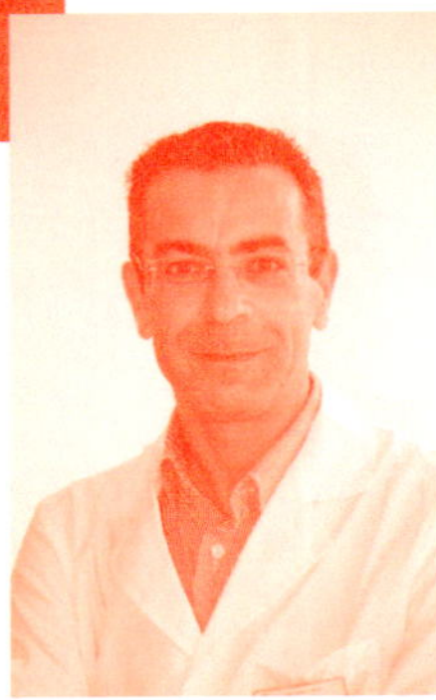
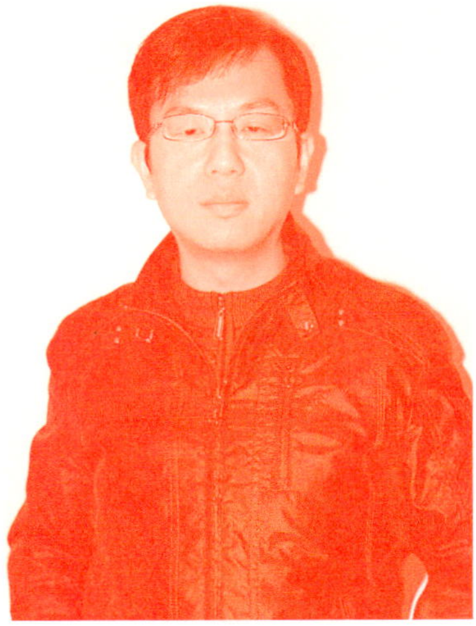
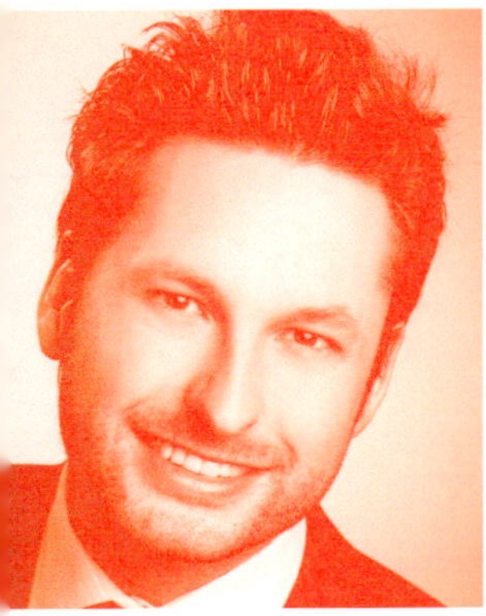
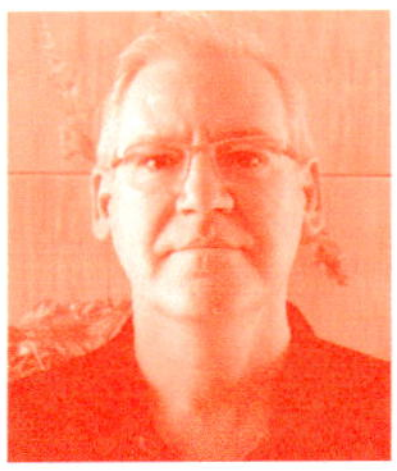

IntechOpen

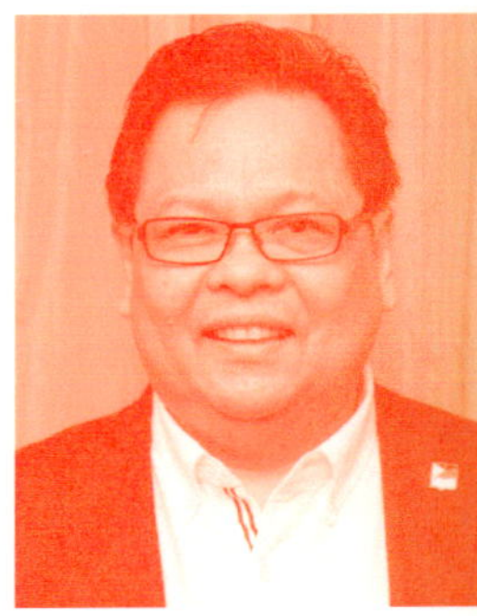
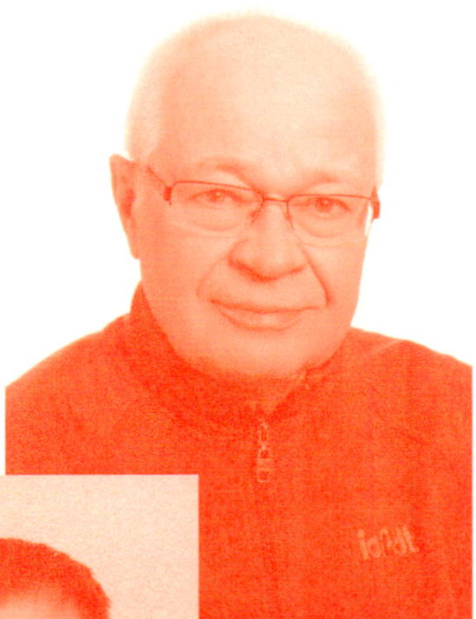
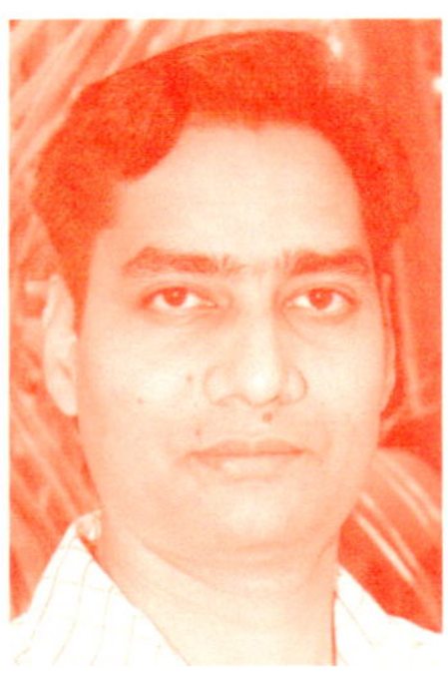
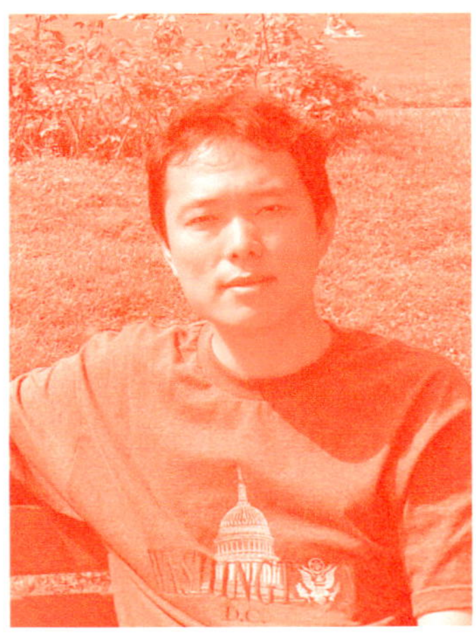
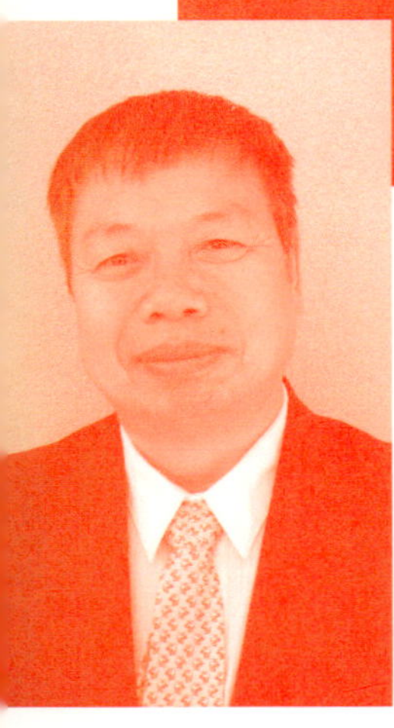
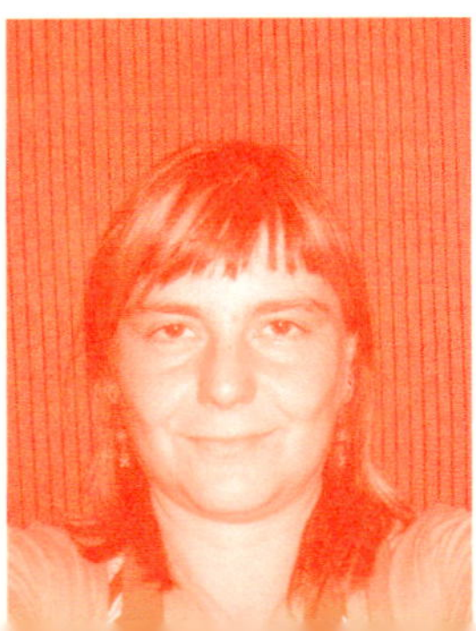

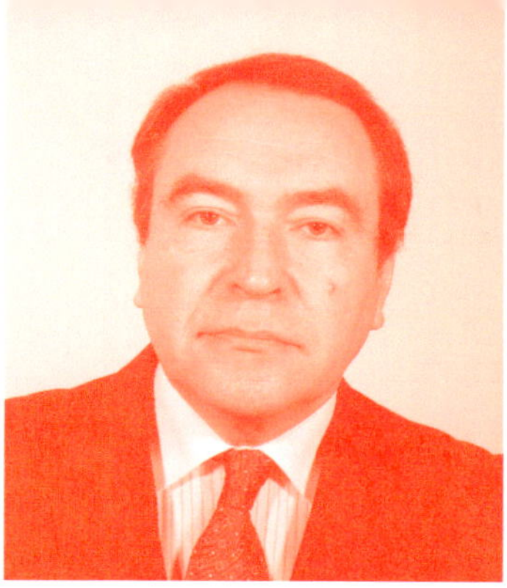

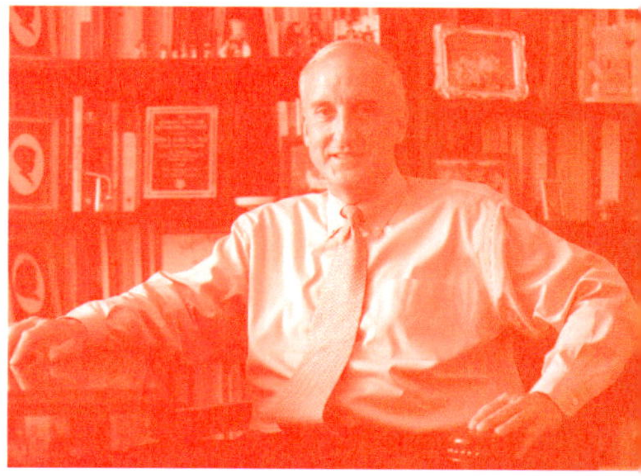

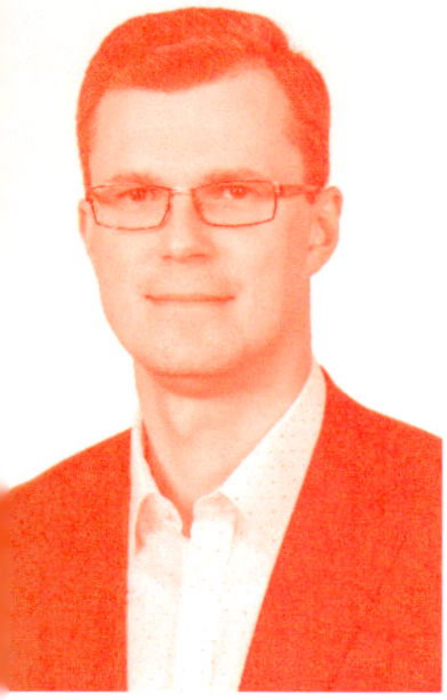

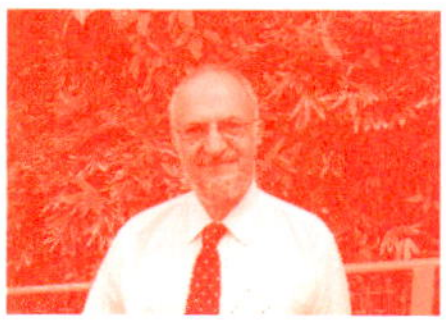

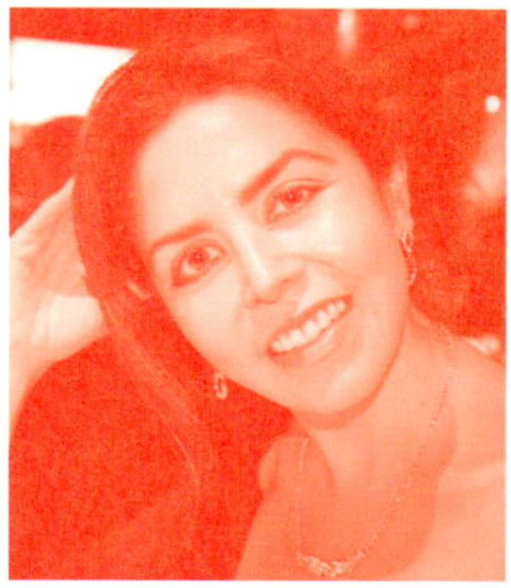

Supporting open minds since 2005

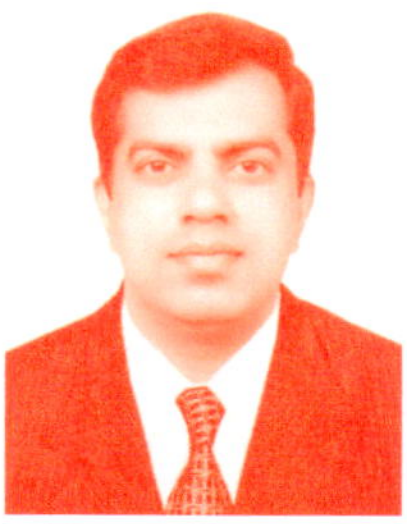

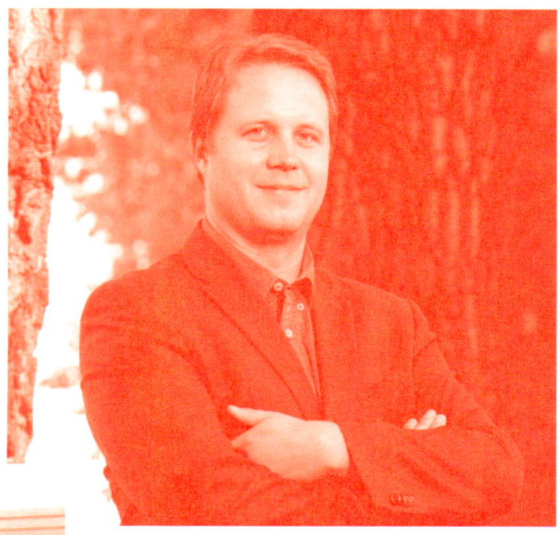

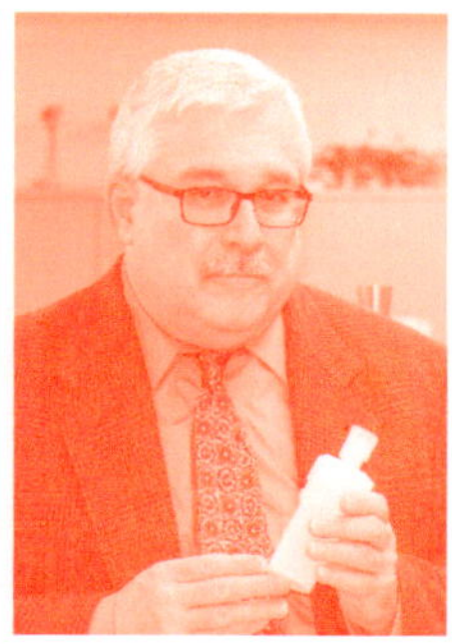

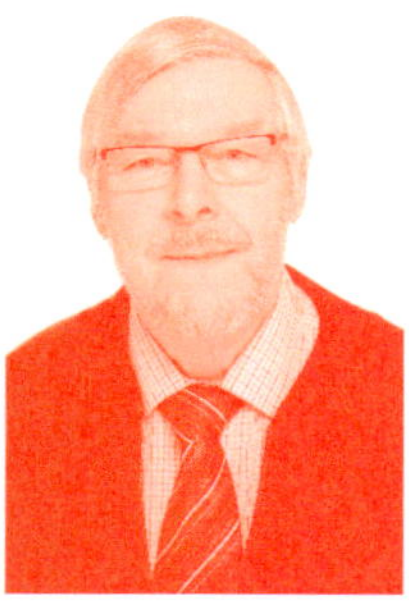

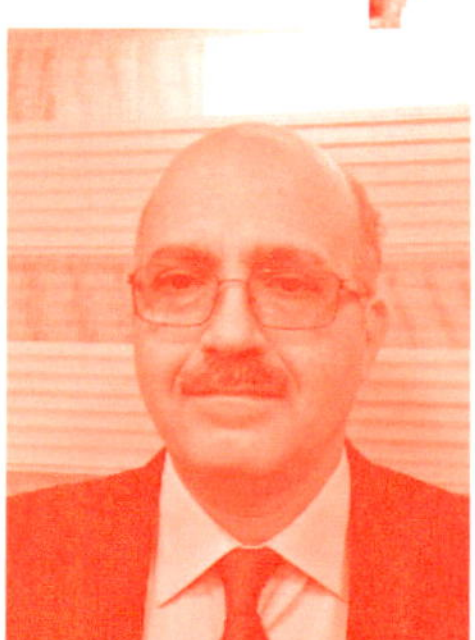

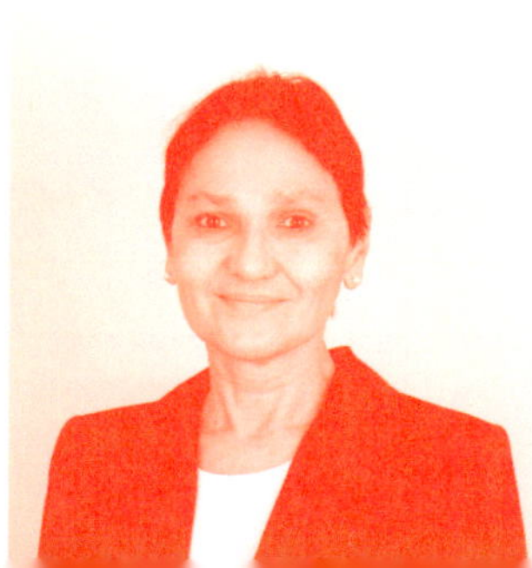

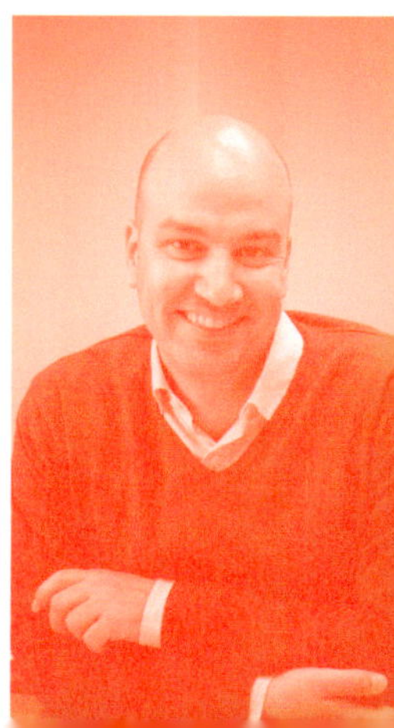

Surgical Recovery
http://dx.doi.org/10.5772/intechopen.77766
Edited by Selim Sozen

Contributors
Michael E. Hantes, George Paraskevas Chalatsis, George Bakagiannis, Sohel Mohamed Gamal Ahmed, Malek Ahmad Alali, Kathy Lynn Gaviola Atuel, Mogahed Ismail Hassan Hussein, Marta Wroblewska, Beata Sulik-Tyszka, Wojciech Figiel, Krzysztof Zieniewicz, Marta Wróblewska, Domenico Viggiano, Alessandro Gonfiotti, Andrea Droghetti, Leonardo Politi, Hector Cesar Duran Vega, Marcelo Uriarte, Juan Carlos Zambrano Bürgl, Jorge Bayter, Lazaro Cárdenas Camarena, Alejandro Lopez Echaury, Selim Sozen, Burhan Hakan Kanat, Erhan Eröz, Atakan Saçlı, Nizamettin Kutluer, Mehmet Gencturk

First published in London, United Kingdom, 2020 by IntechOpen
IntechOpen is the global imprint of INTECHOPEN LIMITED, registered in England and Wales, registration number: 11086078, 5 Princes Gate Court, London, SW7 2QJ, United Kingdom
Printed in Croatia

British Library Cataloguing-in-Publication Data
A catalogue record for this book is available from the British Library

Additional hard and PDF copies can be obtained from orders@intechopen.com

Surgical Recovery
Edited by Selim Sozen
p. cm.
Print ISBN 978-1-83880-891-4
Online ISBN 978-1-83880-892-1
eBook (PDF) ISBN 978-1-83880-893-8

For EU product safety concerns:
IN TECH d.o.o., Prolaz Marije Krucifikse Kozulić 3, 51000 Rijeka, Croatia, info@intechopen.com or visit our website at intechopen.com.

Meet the editor

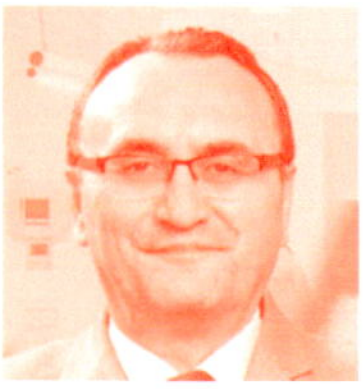

Dr. Selim Sözen was born on 01.01.1973. He graduated from the Faculty of Medicine, Ondokuz Mayıs University, Turkey in 1998. He trained in general surgery at Ankara Atatürk Education and Research Hospital in Turkey (2004). He worked as a specialist at different Government Hospitals in Turkey (2004-2013). He started to work as an Associate Professor at the Department of General Surgery of Medicine Faculty of Namık Kemal University (2013). He completed liver transplantation surgery at İnönü University (General Surgery Department, 2014–2015, Turkey) Fellowship Programs. From 2016, he has worked as a Specialist at his own clinic in İstanbul, Turkey. He is a member of the Turkish Surgical Association. His clinical interests include treatment, surgical procedures, surgical techniques, laparoscopic surgery, minimally invasive surgery, gastrointestinal surgery, hernia surgery, colorectal surgery, surgical oncology, hepatopancreatobilliary surgery, bariatric surgery for morbid obesity, bariatric medicine, endocrine surgery, esophageal diseases, breast surgery, and esophagectomy. Dr Sözen is an author of 93 publications including 3 book chapters, as well as a member of review boards of several journals.

Contents

Preface

One year ago I was kindly asked by editorial consultants at IntechOpen (www.intechweb.org), leading Open Access publisher of scientific books and journals in the science, technology, and medicine fields; to edit a book that would provide comprehensive knowledge on surgical recovery. I was also asked to write the preface for this book, which I am delighted to do. The invitation itself brought up a few questions. What should the style and structure of the book be? Should it be in the form of a textbook or handbook, whereby the titles of chapters reflect a fundamental structure and the content of the educational book or should it be a collection of selected comprehensive review articles, reports of original studies, and case presentations? We ended up with the kind of book that can be characterized as a collection of review papers mainly on surgical recovery, and a few golden pieces of original research. In this context I think that the fact that the 28 authors of the papers work in different countries and institutions amplified the value of their shared reviews, opinions, and unique clinical and pathological experience. A reader of the book, therefore, will be able to find essential knowledge and key facts about postoperative care and surgical recovery.

In the first part, Dr. Sohel Ahmed et al. reminded us of the ASA classification and its importance. The second paper, “ERAS in general thoracic surgery” written by Domenico Viggiano et al.(Italy), was dedicated to the management of the ERAS protocol. Enhanced recovery after surgery (ERAS) is a strategy that seeks to reduce patients’ perioperative stress response, thereby reducing potential complications, decreasing hospital length of stay and enabling patients to return more quickly to their baseline functional status. “Single-row versus Double-row repair in rotator cuff tears” (Hantes Michael E, Greece) covers a rotator cuff (RC) tear. This chapter focuses on differences between two techniques regarding biomechanics, clinical results, healing rate and cost effectiveness. Héctor Durán (México) explores the most important aspects of body contouring surgery. The areas to be improved are nutritional, immunological, pain and inflammation, hemodynamic, early mobilization, patient education and communication, and leadership to evaluate if it has been completed correctly. The overview “Surgical recovery of intestinal obtructions: Pre and postoperative care and how could it be prevented?” (written by Selim Sözen and co-workers, Turkey) draws limits and shows the significance of the surgical management of intestinal obstruction. In the last chapter, Marta Wróblewska (Poland) reminds us of the importance of infection in transplant patients.

I am pleased to see this book on surgical recovery. I salute the authors for their professional dedication and outstanding work in summarizing their clinical and research practices.

Selim Sözen
Associate Professor of General Surgery,
Sözen Surgery Clinic,
İstanbul, Turkey

Section 1

Anesthesia and Surgery

Chapter 1

American Society of Anesthesiologists Physical Status Classification System: History, Development, Reliability, and Its Future

Sohel M.G. Ahmed, Malek Ahmad Alali, Kathy Lynn Gaviola Atuel and Mogahed Ismail Hassan Hussein

Abstract

The American Society of Anesthesiologists Physical Status (ASA PS) classification has long been used as a ranking system that quantifies patient health before anaesthesia and surgery. When initially developed, the ASA PS intended application was purely statistical. However, nowadays it is commonly used by surgical specialties to determine a patient's likelihood of developing postoperative complications, despite studies reporting scoring method subjectivity and inconsistencies among anaesthesiologists in assigning these scores. Over the years, the ASA PS classifications have undergone many changes and modifications to address its limitations. There are a few points to be discussed if all shortcomings are to be treated and interobserver variability is to be limited.

Keywords: American, society, anaesthesiologists, physical, status, classification

1. History

A practising anaesthesiologist will understand the fear exhibited by patients receiving anaesthesia, but fortunately, death from anaesthesia has reduced dramatically with the emergence of modern anaesthesia practice [1]. The development of anaesthesia drugs and monitoring and the evolving anaesthesia training have increased anaesthesia safety, especially for patients who are free of comorbidities. This reduction of mortality was first published by the Institute of Medicine (IOM) in the report *To Err Is Human*: they mentioned that death from anaesthesia has decreased from 2 deaths per 10,000 anaesthetics administered in the 1980s to about 1 death per 200,000 to 300,000 anaesthetics administered at the beginning of the twenty-first century [2–4].

Whenever anaesthesia-related death is considered, the American Society of Anesthesiologists Physical Status classification (ASA PS) is mentioned. It is the most commonly used tool by practising anaesthesiologist in the preoperative assessment of patients. This extensive use is owed to its simplicity and seniority. The American Society of Anesthesiologists (ASA) introduced the ASA PS back in 1941 [5]. During that period, the common practice was to classify patients according to their operative risk, but the vision of the ASA committee has helped them to appreciate the complexity of the situation; they admitted that estimating postoperative mortality using preoperative data is a statistically challenging situation, so they have changed

Class	Definition	Examples
I	No organic pathology or patient in whom the pathological process is localised and does not cause any systemic disturbance or abnormality	Fractures without: shock, blood loss, emboli or systemic signs of injury Congenital deformities without systemic disturbance Localised infection without fever Osseous deformities Uncomplicated hernias Any type of operation may fall in this class since only the patient's physical condition is considered
II	A moderate but definite systemic disturbance caused either by the condition that is to be treated by surgical intervention or by other existing pathological processes	Mild diabetes Function capacity I or IIa Psychotic patients unable to care for themselves Mild acidosis Moderate anaemia Septic or acute pharyngitis Acute sinusitis Superficial infection that causes a systemic reaction. Non-toxic thyroid adenoma with all but partial respiratory obstruction Mild thyrotoxicosis
III	Severe systemic disturbance from any cause or causes. It is not possible to state an absolute measure of severity, as this is a matter of clinical judgement	Complicated or severe diabetes Functional capacity IIb Combination of heart and lung diseases that severely impair function Complete intestinal obstruction with serious physiological disturbance Pulmonary tuberculosis causing tachycardia or dyspnoea Prolonged illness with weakness of all or several systems
IV	Extreme systemic disorders which have already become an imminent threat to life regardless of treatment. Due to their duration or nature, there has already been damage to the organism that is irreversible. This class is intended to include only patients who are in extremely poor physical state	Functional capacity III – (cardiac decompensation) Severe trauma with irreparable damage Complete intestinal obstruction in a previously debilitated patient Cardiovascular disease with marked renal impairment Anaesthesia to arrest marked blood loss from secondary haemorrhage in a patient in poor condition
V	Emergencies that would be otherwise graded as Class 1 or 2	
VI	Emergencies that would otherwise be graded as Class 3–4	

Table 1.
ASA PS as described in 1941 [5].

the notion of operative risk into physical status. The purpose of that classification was to create a common platform for doctors to guide the patient classification for further future statistical analysis. There were four classes (**Table 1**), and if there was an emergency surgery, then the class will be five for a patient who was classified as 1–2 and six for a patient who was classified as 3–4. Surgery was considered an emergency whenever the surgeon said so [5]. Clinical scenarios were assigned to each class for easy use. They further added an alphabetic scaling, ranging from A to D according to the objective evidence of cardiovascular decompensation, with A being no evidence and D being severely decompensated (**Table 2**).

After 20 years, some authors removed the clinical scenarios, added a fifth class, and added the letter E to indicate emergencies (**Figure 1**). This change was a result of a large study that was aiming to assess the postoperative motility using preoperative physical status [6].

Retrospectives trials to validate ASA scale have then become numerous added to the many prospective trials, and they gave birth to ASA pooled mortality [7]. In

Class	Objective evidence of cardiovascular disease
A	No objective evidence of cardiovascular disease. No symptoms and no limitation in ordinary physical activity
B	Objective evidence of minimal cardiovascular disease. Mild symptoms and slight limitation during ordinary activity. Comfortable at rest
C	Objective evidence of moderately severe cardiovascular disease. Marked limitation in activity due to symptoms, even during less-than-ordinary activity. Comfortable only at rest
D	Objective evidence of severe cardiovascular disease. Severe limitations. Experiences symptoms even while at rest

Table 2.
Additional clinical classification based on cardiovascular state [5].

Class	Definition	Examples
1	Normal health	Healthy, non-smoking, no or minimal alcohol use
2	Mild systemic disease	Mild diseases only without substantive functional limitations. Examples include (but not limited to): current smoker, social alcohol drinker, pregnancy, 30 < BMI < 40, well-controlled DM/HTN, mild lung disease
3	Severe systemic disease	Substantive functional limitations. One or more moderate to severe diseases. Examples include (but not limited to): poorly controlled DM or HTN, COPD, morbid obesity (BMI ≥ 40), active hepatitis, alcohol dependence or abuse, implanted pacemaker, moderate reduction in ejection fraction, ESRD undergoing regularly scheduled dialysis, premature infant PCA < 60 weeks, history (> 3 months) of MI, CVA, TIA or CAD/stents
4	Severe systemic disease that is a constant threat to life	Examples include (but not limited to): recent (< 3 months) MI, CVA, TIA or CAD/stents, ongoing cardiac ischaemia or severe valve dysfunction, severe reduction in ejection fraction, sepsis, DIC, ARD or ESRD not undergoing regularly scheduled dialysis
5	Moribund: survival not expected without surgery	Examples include (but not limited to): ruptured abdominal/thoracic aneurysm, massive trauma, intracranial bleed with mass effect, ischaemic bowel in the face of significant cardiac pathology or multiple organ/system dysfunction
6	Brain-dead organ donor	

Figure 1.
The latest update on ASA [8].

Physiological variables	Operative variables
Chest Hx	Type of surgery
Age	Severity
Cardiovascular Hx	Number of procedures
ECG	Blood loss
BP	Malignancy
HR	
GCS	
WBC	
Hb	
Urea	
Na+	
K+	

Table 3.
POSSUM variables.

1980 another revision (**Table 3**) was carried out, which resulted in the addition of a new class that considers braindead patients [8].

Although ASA PS is widely used, it appears that no much effort or attention was paid by the researcher to improve this tool until recently when some models considered ASA physical status as a part of their risk assessment system.

2. Risk assessment systems

2.1 The surgical risk scale

The Surgical Risk Scale is a simple tool that was created by the combination of ASA scale and the British United Provident Association (BUPA) along with the Confidential Enquiry into Perioperative Death (NCEPOD). It was tested in a prospective study; they used logistic regression analysis and created a scale ranging from 3 to 14, which is simple and accurate [9].

2.2 The American College of Surgeons National Surgical Quality Improvement Program (ACS NSQIP)

The ACS main idea behind this study was to compare particular risk assessment scores to a universal tool. They provided surgeons with an online application that considers ASA scale. The study results showed that ACS NSQIP variables are significant in ASA scale validation [10].

2.3 The surgical outcome risk tool (SORT)

This risk assessment tool was developed and validated in 2014 in the UK. ASA PS was added along with other six variables: the urgency of surgery, high-risk surgery, severity, age, and the presence of cancer obtained from NCEPOD data analysis [11].

2.4 The National Emergency Laparotomy Audit (NELA) score

As the name implies, it's an audit for more than 50,000 cases. All patients were above 18 years. It was only used to assess mortality inpatient undergoing laparotomy for small bowel obstruction. ASA scale was studied for its association with the patient outcome.

3. Validity

Something is valid when it can fulfil the objective against which it's being tested, and its reliability depends on consistency. Every reliable tool is valid, but not every valid tool is reliable.

In terms of assessing mortality, the ASA scale is not valid by itself, but this is not a discovery; this was first mentioned in the same original paper by ASA committee itself [12]. Assessing the patient physical status is surely what ASA scale is best used for, but here comes the issue of how reliable it is.

Subjectivity in patient assessment is the source of the variability in the scale use.

Many studies have been investigating ASA scale reliability. They either assessed the consistency of the classification of many patients by a specific number of doctors to evaluate the factors associated with inconsistency if found or evaluated the classification of particular cases among doctors. Effective studies to assess the statistical validity of the scale started to appear 20 years after the original scale was described [6]. Studies to determine the reliability of the scale by assessing its consistency only begun in the late 1970s [13]. In 1978 a questionnaire was developed and was emailed to more than 200 anaesthesiologists to test how consistent is ASA scale in the classification of 10 imaginary clinical scenarios (**Figure 2**). They reported a consistency rate of 5.9, which was affected by whether the anaesthesiologist was doing a private or academic work and with no effect of the region of practice [13]. Age, history of ischemic heart disease, abnormal BMI, and low haemoglobin level appeared to be where conflicts arise. Many years after a study found that there is no significant correlation between expertise in anaesthesia and scale reliability [14]. A more recent study confirmed that result and showed the absence of a relationship between the scale reliability and the age, level of training, or how expert the anaesthesiologist is [15].

The association between the accuracy of scale and whether the user is an anaesthesiologist or not appeared to be significant [16]. Some recent studies claimed that the removal of clinical scenarios affected the scale reliability; they consider it to be a self-correcting tool that empowers the system [17, 12].

Patient 4

A 42-year-old Negro man is scheduled for a lumbar laminectomy for a herniated disc at L2–3. Past history and review of systems reveal a previous diagnosis of sickle-cell trait. The rest of the history is noncontributory. Physical examination shows no abnormality except neurologic findings compatible with the herniated lumbar disc.

Hemoglobin is 11.8 g/100 ml and hematocrit, 36.4 per cent.

Figure 2.
Example of a clinical scenario used for the validation [13].

4. Alternatives

Stop your flow of thoughts for a moment. Now think of this question, what is the main aim of medical care? Many doctors will say that it depends on the specialty. That is partially correct because there is a common place where all doctors meet along the road of patient care, which is to alleviate the patient suffering. So we are not fighting death, and we want to make sure that the patient is not going to die from a preventable cause and is not going to suffer from a bad quality of life. Reducing avoidable mortality along with the people who desire to know their chances of being alive after undergoing surgery has motivated doctors from specialties that are concerned with the preoperative assessment of patients to develop many tools and scales to assess the expected patient mortality.

For us to talk about the possible alternative scores for ASA physical status scale, we need to point out for what reason the scale was created and what variables were included. ASA introduced the classification system back in 1941 to facilitate the statistical calculation of operative patient risk rather than indicating it. They classified the patients according to their physical status to create a common background for patients sorting by surgeons and anaesthesiologists and then assess the association between different classes and patient outcome. The ASA classification itself does not consider many other important factors that may affect the patient outcome (severity of the surgery, the experience of the surgeon, the quality of the hospitals, etc.) [5]. So in terms of patient sorting function, ASA classification is standing on the top if not alone with only a mild problem of subjectivity. But in mortality assessment, it can only be a part of bigger scales, as the pooled mortality for ASA grades obtained using clinical audits was found to be increased with many other factors like intraoperative blood loss, duration of the operation, and in-hospital mortality [7].

There are many scores to predict patient mortality after surgery or in specific conditions. In this chapter, we will only review nonselective scores that predict mortality in surgical patients.

4.1 ASA pooled mortality

After the ASA was being revised into five classes in 1961 [18], many retrospective studies have shown a link between ASA classes and perioperative mortality rate [19–22]. The first prospective study to determine the correlation between ASA classification, perioperative risks, and postoperative outcome with a large number of patients was in 1996. They assigned patients with all types of surgery, and they have taken into account the type of surgery, patient lab results, perioperative risk variables, time of the operation, and the type of anaesthesia. They used univariate analysis and logistic regression analysis to estimate the mortality rate (**Figure 3**) for each ASA class [7].

ASA class	Definition	Pooled mortality (%)
I	Healthy	0–0.3
II	Mild systemic disease with no functional limitation	0.3–1.4
III	Severe systemic disease with functional limitation	1.8–5.4
IV	Severe systemic disease – constant threat to life	7.8–25.0
V	Moribund patient – unlikely to survive 24 h with or without operation	9.4–57.8
E	Suffix added to denote emergency operation	

Figure 3.
ASA pooled mortality.

4.2 Physiological and operative severity score for the enumeration of mortality and morbidity (POSSUM)

This is a risk assessment tool that uses both physiological and operative factors into account (**Table 3**). A prospective study of 10,000 surgical interventions except for paediatric surgery and day-case surgery, applying logistic regression analysis, showed that the POSSUM equation overestimates mortality [23]. A further modification of POSSUM, which was named P-POSSUM, was found to be more accurate in mortality prediction [23].

4.3 Preoperative score to predict postoperative mortality (POSPOM)

A very large cohort study for 1 year was conducted in France. Seventeen variables were used to estimate the mortality risk for 2,717,902 patients. The risk tool was validated by using the logistic model.

4.4 Frailty scores

Assessing frailty in the elderly has become an evolving practice of the twenty-first century. Validated frailty criteria (weakness, fatigue, decreased physical activity, and walking speed), also known as frailty phenotype, were the result of a cohort study that used the cardiovascular health study database. Two cohorts were randomised in 1989, and they were followed for 4 to 7 years [24]. Another model that exists in the literature is the frailty index, which is the impact of frailty detected during geriatric assessment [25]. Notice that each criterion has its particular measurement consideration, and it is not discussed as it is beyond the scope of this chapter. Many studies have used these criteria to assess postoperative mortality in different pathologies [26–28].

5. Comparison of systems

Many studies have explored the issue of which the scale is superior to others, but we have to keep in mind that many variables will be adjusted to make the comparison possible, and this is mainly because of the broad variability between these scores and the different objectives and settings at which each score was introduced.

To understand this in a better way, we must understand the meaning of risk in anaesthesia. Risk indicates the negative impact of a process which may be started in the past, may be happening now, or is probably going to occur in the future. Human survival nature is evident in the efforts that we put on trying to reduce all the risks.

For every patient undergoing surgery, four broad risk categories can be faced:

1. Hospital hazard.

2. Risk of anaesthesia.

3. Surgery.

4. Patient factors.

The ASA PS focuses only on patient status and the risk of anaesthesia; POSPOM, POSSUM, and P-POSSUM have an additional focus on surgical risk. But every score assesses the same variable differently because this is affected by the use of the tool in practice; as ASA is the standard practice for years, then it will have the upper arm in assessing patient factors. None of them considered hospital hazard. The ASA itself varies on its validity between its different versions. The original ASA used to have clinical scenarios that approximate the subjective variations between doctors, which were removed from the updated versions. The authors of the study that introduced and validated POSPOM in 2016 claimed that ASA PS is a deficient tool for assessing mortality risk because it does not take risks apart from patient factors and anaesthesia risk into account [29]. Many retrospective and prospective studies have studied ASA PS correlation with mortality after considering all the other elements, and many other trails have tackled the issue off subjectivity and figured to solve it with a robust statistical methodology many years before 2016 [7, 30].

This risk assessment issue can be solved with a meeting that involves public health, anaesthesia, surgery, and medical statistic expertise to create an assessment tool that considers all these risks and to be statistically applicable and clinically standardised to avoid subjectivity.

Author details

Sohel M.G. Ahmed[1]*, Malek Ahmad Alali[1], Kathy Lynn Gaviola Atuel[1] and Mogahed Ismail Hassan Hussein[2]

1 Department of Anaesthesia and Perioperative Medicine, Hamad Medical Corporation, Doha, Qatar

2 Faculty of Medicine, University of Gezira, Sudan

*Address all correspondence to: sohelm@yahoo.com

References

[1] Cooper JB, Gaba D. No myth: Anesthesia is a model for addressing patient safety. Anesthesiology. 2002; **97**(6):1335-1337

[2] Cranshaw J, Gupta KJ, Cook TM. Litigation related to drug errors in anaesthesia: An analysis of claims against the NHS in England 1995–2007. Anaesthesia. 2009;**64**(12): 1317-1323

[3] Lagasse RS. Anesthesia safety: Model or myth? Anesthesiology. 2002;**97**(6): 1609-1617

[4] To Err Is Human, Washington. D.C.: National Academies Press; 2000

[5] Uwe K. Grading patients for surgical procedures. Anesthesiology. 1941;**31**(4): 305-309

[6] Dripps RD, Lamont A, Eckenhoff JE. The role of anesthesia in surgical mortality. JAMA. 1961;**178**(3):261

[7] Wolters U, Wolf T, Stützer H, Schröder T. ASA classification and perioperative variables as predictors of postoperative outcome. British Journal of Anaesthesia. 1996;**77**(2):217-222

[8] Fitz-Henry J. The ASA classification and peri-operative risk. Annals of the Royal College of Surgeons of England. 2011;**93**(3):185-187

[9] Sutton R, Bann S, Brooks M, Sarin S. The surgical risk scale as an improved tool for risk-adjusted analysis in comparative surgical audit. The British Journal of Surgery. 2002;**89**(6):763-768

[10] Bilimoria KY et al. Development and evaluation of the universal ACS NSQIP surgical risk calculator: A decision aid and informed consent tool for patients and surgeons. Journal of the American College of Surgeons. 2013; **217**(5):833-842.e3

[11] Protopapa KL, Simpson JC, Smith NCE, Moonesinghe SR. Development and validation of the surgical outcome risk tool (SORT). The British Journal of Surgery. Dec. 2014; **101**(13):1774-1783

[12] Mayhew D, Mendonca V, Murthy BVS. A review of ASA physical status—Historical perspectives and modern developments. Anaesthesia. 2019;**74**(3):373-379

[13] Owens WD, Felts JA, Spitznagel EL. ASA physical status classifications. Anesthesiology. 1978;**49**(4):239-243

[14] Haynes SR, Lawler PGP. An assessment of the consistency of ASA physical status classification allocation. Anaesthesia. 1995;**50**(3):195-199

[15] Riley RH, Holman CDJ, Fletcher DR. Inter-rater reliability of the ASA physical status classification in a sample of anaesthetists in Western Australia. Anaesthesia and Intensive Care. 2014; **42**(5):614-618

[16] Curatolo C, Goldberg A, Maerz D, Lin HM, Shah H, Trinh M. ASA physical status assignment by non-anesthesia providers: Do surgeons consistently downgrade the ASA score preoperatively? Journal of Clinical Anesthesia. 2017;**38**:123-128

[17] Hurwitz EE et al. Adding examples to the ASA-physical status classification improves correct assignment to patients. Anesthesiology. Apr. 2017;**126**(4): 614-622

[18] Dripps. New classification of physical status. Anesthesiology. 1961;**24**: 111

[19] Farrow SC, Fowkes FGR, Lunn JN, Robertson IB, Samuel P. Epidemiology in anesthesia II: Factors affecting

mortality in hospitals. British Journal of Anaesthesia. 1982;**54**(8):811-817

[20] Pedersen T et al. Risk factors, complications and outcome in anaesthesia. A pilot study. European Journal of Anaesthesiology. May 1986; **3**(3):225-239

[21] Marx GF, Mateo CV, Orkin LR. Computer analysis of postanesthetic deaths. Anesthesiology. Jul. 1973;**39**(1): 54-58

[22] Vacanti CJ, VanHouten RJ, Hill RC. A statistical analysis of the relationship of physical status to postoperative mortality in 68,388 cases. Anesthesia & Analgesia. 1970;**49**(4):564-566

[23] Peacock O et al. Thirty-day mortality in patients undergoing laparotomy for small bowel obstruction. The British Journal of Surgery. Jul. 2018; **105**(8):1006-1013

[24] Fried LP et al. Frailty in older adults: Evidence for a phenotype. The Journals of Gerontology. Series A, Biological Sciences and Medical Sciences. Mar. 2001;**56**(3):M146-M156

[25] Chen X, Mao G, Leng SX. Frailty syndrome: An overview. Clinical Interventions in Aging. 2014;**9**:433-441

[26] McGuckin DG, Mufti S, Turner DJ, Bond C, Moonesinghe SR. The association of peri-operative scores, including frailty, with outcomes after unscheduled surgery. Anaesthesia. 2018; **73**(7):819-824

[27] Makary MA et al. Frailty as a predictor of surgical outcomes in older patients. Journal of the American College of Surgeons. 2010;**210**(6): 901-908

[28] Kim S et al. Multidimensional frailty score for the prediction of postoperative mortality risk. JAMA Surgery. 2014; **149**(7):633

[29] Le Manach Y et al. Preoperative score to predict postoperative mortality (POSPOM). Anesthesiology. 2016; **124**(3):570-579

[30] Davenport DL, Bowe EA, Henderson WG, Khuri SF, Mentzer RM. National Surgical Quality Improvement Program (NSQIP) risk factors can be used to validate American Society of Anesthesiologists Physical Status Classification (ASA PS) levels. Annals of Surgery. 2006;**243**(5):636-644

Section 2

Enhanced Recovery After Surgery (ERAS)

Chapter 2

ERAS in General Thoracic Surgery

Domenico Viggiano, Leonardo Politi, Alessandro Gonfiotti and Andrea Droghetti

Abstract

Enhanced recovery after surgery (ERAS®) is a strategy that seeks to reduce patients' perioperative stress response, thereby reducing potential complications, decreasing hospital length of stay and enabling patients to return more quickly to their baseline functional status. This programme results from the union of several perioperative clinical elements that have individually proved to be beneficial to the patient and have showed, when used together, a synergy that results in a significant outcome improvement. The term was coined at the end of the 1990s and originally used to refer to a complex fast-track programme in open colorectal surgery. Subsequently, the practice has spread to other surgical specialties centralising the interest of clinicians and researchers. The objective of this chapter is to analyse the key elements of an ERAS protocol applicable to minimally invasive thoracic surgery.

Keywords: ERAS, fast track, VATS lobectomy, lung cancer, surgical recovery

1. Introduction

ERAS is the acronym of enhanced recovery after surgery: a multimodal perioperative approach based on the best medical evidence [1]. This programme results from the union of several perioperative clinical elements that have individually proved to be beneficial to the patient and have showed, when used together, a synergy that results in a significant outcomes improvement.

The key elements of each ERAS protocol include preoperative counselling and nutrition, avoidance of perioperative fasting and carbohydrate loading up to 2 h preoperatively, standardised anaesthetic and analgesic regimens (epidural and non-opioid analgesia) and early mobilisation (**Figure 1**) [2]. A meta-analysis showed that ERAS programmes in major surgery reduce hospitalisation by 2–3 days and complications by 30–50% [3].

From its introduction at the start of 1990s, ERAS has improved perioperative approach of many specialities: general surgery (colon resection) [4], vascular surgery [5], thoracic surgery [6, 7] and recently urology (cystectomy) [8, 9]. The aim of such programmes is to try to change the physiological and psychological responses to major surgery [1]: the experiences collected until now have shown a reduction in complications and hospital stay, improvements in cardiopulmonary function, earlier return of bowel function and earlier resumption of normal activities [10, 11].

There are relatively few reports on the use of ERAS in thoracic surgery; the aim of our paper is to focus on the key elements of an ERAS protocol, evaluating their applicability in thoracic surgery oncology, particularly in the field of minimally invasive surgery.

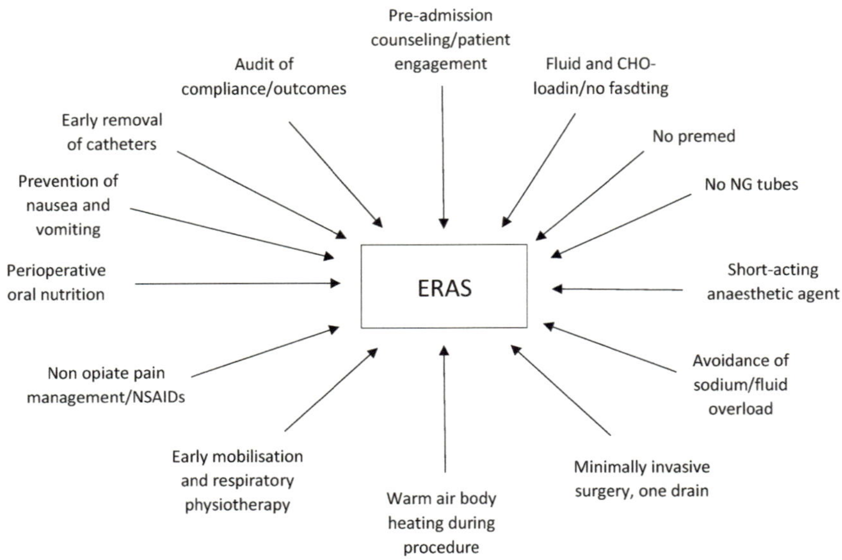

Figure 1.
The key elements of ERAS protocol.

2. Principles of ERAS

Response to major surgery is inevitable: for many years, this was a postulate in conventional perioperative metabolic care. This concept has recently been challenged with the view that a substantial element of the stress response can be avoided with the appropriate application of modern anaesthetic, analgesic and metabolic support techniques. Another referral point in conventional post-operative care was the patient's prolonged bed rest: this concept is now under revision also [12]. In the catabolic patient, medium-term functional decline will ensue if active steps are not taken to return the patient to full function as soon as possible. Based on these two concepts, a new view of peri-operative surgical care has been created, based on the principles of stress reduction and promotion of return to baseline after surgery, avoiding medium term sequelae of conventional post-operative care (e.g. loss in

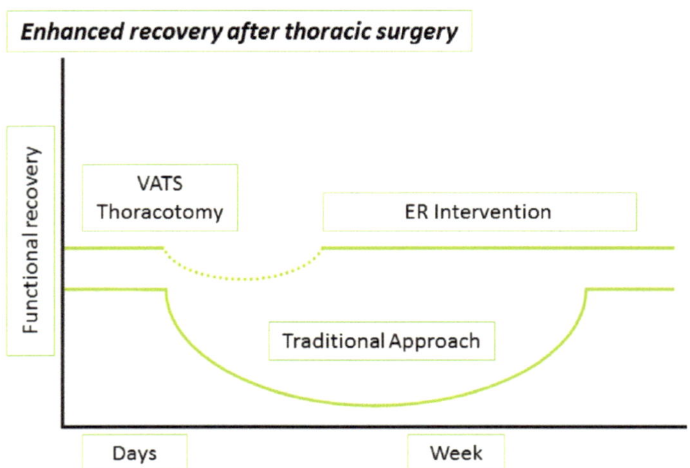

Figure 2.
Multidisciplinary approach to the ERAS protocol.

nutritional status and fatigue) [13]. So, the ERAS programme results in a clinical pathway with the aim of attenuate surgical stress, maintain physiological function and expedite return to normal function; a cornerstone of each ERAS protocol is a real multidisciplinary approach, avoiding the so-called silo mentality, defined as 'an attitude found in some organisations that occurs when several departments or groups do not want to share information or knowledge with other individuals in the same company' [14] (**Figure 2**).

3. ERAS key elements

3.1 Preadmission counselling and patient information

It is well known that an exhaustive preoperative patient information can enhance post-operative recovery and pain relief, particularly in patients who show most denial and the highest levels of anxiety [15, 16] **Figure 1**. A clear and comprehensible explanation of what is to happen during a patient's hospital stay can also facilitate adherence to the care pathway and allows timely recovery and an early discharge: patients should receive oral and written preadmission information forms describing what will happen during their hospital stay, what they have to expect, and what will be their role during their recovery. In addition, at the first meeting, the patient should also be given a specific role with clear tasks to perform during the post-operative period [17]. These include targets for food intakes and oral nutritional supplements (ONS) and targets for staying out of bed.

3.2 Preoperative fasting and metabolic condition

Fasting after midnight has been the standard in elective surgery to avoid pulmonary aspiration without obtaining scientific support: a recent review [18] has shown that this practice is not only not useful but, in some cases, even negative for the patient's metabolism. Current recommendations from leading national anaesthesia society suggest clear fluid intake up to 2 h from anaesthesia induction and a 6-h fast for solid foods [19–21]. Some works in the literature, which analysed the effects of preoperative fasting on patients, concluded by proposing that patients arrive in the operating theatre fed. Examples of preoperative nutrition are the use of clear carbohydrate-rich beverages (12.6%) at a dose of 800 ml before midnight and 400 ml 2–3 h before surgery: this leads to a reduction in thirst, hunger and anxiety in patients awaiting surgery [22] and to a significant reduction in post-operative insulin resistance [23]. In this way, the patients' metabolism benefits more from post-operative nutrition [24] with a lower risk of hyperglycaemia [25]. This approach, validated for different major surgery, is easy to apply also for thoracic surgery.

3.3 Anaesthetic protocol and multimodal pain relief

According to ERAS principles, the efforts of anaesthetic procedure has to be made to minimise the impact of anaesthetic agents and techniques on organ function and also to ensure appropriate depth of anaesthesia and avoidance of awareness but also avoiding overdose: it is rational, therefore, to use agents with short pharmacodynamic duration (propofol and remifentanil) [26], thereby allowing pro-active recovery to start on the day of surgery. Thus, opioids with longer-lasting effect (morphine and fentanyl) should be avoided. Short acting inhalation anaesthesia is a reasonable alternative to total intravenous anaesthesia. Although the protective role of epidural analgesia before the beginning of surgery, by limiting the production of stress hormones and post-operative insulin resistance, has been sufficiently clarified, its effect on post-operative outcome is still debated [27]. Epidural analgesia has been identified for usual post-operative analgesia because of its optimal pain relief capacity and the benefits on post-operative [28]. However, a recent large single study [29] has questioned the benefits of epidural analgesia in terms of post-operative morbidity and mortality. Moreover, it is necessary to take into account the risks associated with the procedure: epidural hematomas, abscesses or neurological damage are in the order of 0.01–0.6 [30]. The catheter is positioned in the awake patient to establish the effectiveness of the block. During surgery, the block can be maintained by continuous infusion of local anaesthetic (e.g. bupivacaine 0.1%) plus a low-dose opiate (e.g. 2 mg/ml fentanyl) at 4–10 ml/h. Epidural opioids in small does synergise with epidural local anaesthetics in providing analgesia, allowing a reduced dosage of both agents. Furthermore, low-dose epidural opioids improve the analgesic effects without major systemic effects [31]. Finally, it has been demonstrated that the addition of a small dose of adrenaline to epidural infusion of local anaesthetic and opioid enhances the analgesic effect of these drugs avoiding systemic opioid related side-effects [32–34].

Analysing the data presented in the literature of recent controlled studies and a Cochrane review, several studies [35] highlight how early mobilisation is effectively obtained using continuous epidural local anaesthetic or local anaesthetic-opioid techniques. Epidural local anaesthetic techniques provide a more effective analgesia than patient controlled analgesia (PCA), allowing greater physiological benefits on surgical stress responses; achieving the randomised studies have demonstrated that continuous epidural analgesia has positive effects on the reduction of pulmonary morbidity, but not on other types of morbidity or on hospital stay and convalescence [36]. This probably for unimodal intervention that does not take advantage of the efficient analgesia: the use of non-steroid anti-inflammatory drugs (NSAIDs) may provide some additional analgesia [37]. The principal objective for post-operative analgesia is eliminating opioid with their opioid-related side effects and improving quality of recovery [38]. An optimal deadline for post-operative continuous epidural analgesia has not been established; however, 2 days is the period identified from several large case series and normally used in clinical practice. It should also be emphasised that there is no evidence for the use of NSAIDs to improve analgesia in addition to a well-functioning epidural: this practice should be avoided.

There are several papers in the literature that have demonstrated the efficacy of these analgesic principles also for thoracic surgery; for example: the use of epidural analgesia that reduces post-operative morbidity or the use of lower doses of opioid to reduce their adverse effects and promote early mobilisation [39].

3.4 Surgical aspects

Minimally invasive surgery is a central point of any fast-track programme: when applied it has shown its effectiveness in terms of reduction of hospital stay, post-operative complications and pain both in the comparison of VATS surgery vs. open surgery [40] and for standard multiportal VATS vs. uniportal [41]. The comparison between multiportal VATS and uniportal has showed many advantages in favour of the latter: less trauma tissue, less blood loss and less complication. This can potentially be translated into a reduction in post-operative hospitalisation and faster recovery of the daily activities of patients, which is the goal of the ERAS programme. A recent meta-analysis published by Harris and The Collaborative Research (CORE) Group, Macquarie University, Sydney, Australia, compares eight observational studies published over the past two years comparing the outcome of oncologic patients [41] treated with conventional VATS lobectomy (multiport) vs. uniportal VATS. The results (1850 patients, of which 627 treated with uniportal VATS and 1223 with multiportal VATS), show statistically significant differences in favour of the single-port in terms of length of stay (6.2 ± 2.6 vs. 6.7 ± 3.4 days, $P < 0.0001$), duration of thoracic drainage (4.5 ± 2.2 vs. 5.4 ± 2.9 days, $P = 0.0006$), post-operative complications (12.0 vs. 13.7%, $P = 0.009$). Post-operative pain also appeared to be minor in monoportal procedures although with non-statistically significant values. However, taking into account VATS interventions for minor surgery, further work confirms a reduction in post-operative pain using a smaller number of thoracoscopic accesses [42, 43]: in this way appear to be clear a rationale link behind the fewer accesses to the chest and hence fewer intercostal nerves that can be traumatised during surgical procedures.

3.4.1 Minimal invasiveness of VATS approach

The minimal invasiveness of VATS procedures is based on the lower impact of its surgical trauma compared to traditional open procedures by thoracotomy. However, several VATS techniques have been described over the years, differing mainly on the number of ports and their location. The number of ports can be discussed as a factor affecting the invasiveness of the surgical procedure and consequently influencing the post-operative functional recovery. Several authors have highlighted how the transition from VATS multiportal approach to a monoportal approach is effective in optimising post-surgical results by reducing pain, complications and the length of hospital stay. Hence the idea that, in order to optimise surgery within an ERAS programme, monoportal VATS can facilitate a faster recovery of the patient, an early discharge and a promptly return to daily life. Tamura recent study [44] has shown how single-port technique reduces post-operative pain and increases quality of life in the peri-operative period. In two subsequent publications, Rocco and others [42] and Gonfiotti et al. [43] showed that a monoportal VATS approach is less associated with residual pain and post-operative paraesthesia. With the limits of non-randomised observational studies, we believe that these data can allow us to hypothesise that a lesser surgical trauma on the chest wall can result in a faster functional recovery, even when we talk about minimally invasive surgery.

3.4.2 Prevention of post-operative air leak

The air passage from the lung parenchyma into the pleural space after pulmonary resection is called air leak. In the literature, we can find the definition of prolonged air loss (PAL) as an air passage beyond the five post-operative days. Different studies show that the effects of this complication on the post-operative course significantly impacts on the risk of other complications (e.g. pleural empyema), post-operative hospitalisation and increased hospital costs and, more generally, a worse post-operative course.

Prolonged air leak appears to be a rather frequent complication after VATS lobectomy. In the reports of the Italian VATS group the incidence of PAL after a pulmonary lobectomy is equal to 7.2%, similar to the data present in the literature. Therefore, the prevention of a PAL is a fundamental element in ERAS perspective [45, 46]. In addition to this, Brunelli [47] reported a higher rate of pleural empyema in patients with PAL and Varela [48, 49] showed an increased incidence of pneumonia, atelectasis due to sputum retention and pleural effusion, demonstrating how PAL is associated with an increased risk of post-operative complications.

Therefore, it is fundamental to prevent the onset of PAL, mainly by adopting two different strategies:

a. Reduction of residual pleural space

b. Reinforcing/protecting suture line

In a recent paper [50] which considers five selected studies, in four of these, the fissureless technique used in pulmonary lobectomy has shown itself superior to the standard approach for PAL prevention and the reduction of the cessation of air loss time, concluding that, based on the current data, we can consider the fissureless technique better than the standard one [51]. Criticisms of this conclusion are mainly made when considering lower lobectomies: although the fissureless technique is accepted in upper or middle lobectomies, it is not considered as valid for lower lobectomies, mainly for oncological reasons as it could reduce the effectiveness of VATS lymph node dissection of stations N1 [52].

3.4.3 Number of pleural drainages

According to fast-tracking, could be indicated the positioning of just one pleural drainage (28/30 Fr) for all surgical procedure, instead of two used for example after a pulmonary lobectomy; a second drainage tube may be useful when a significant post-operative air leak is expected or in case of a bi-lobectomy [53]. The advantages of positioning a single thoracic drain reside in the reduction of post-operative pain that allows early patient mobilisation and therefore faster recovery [54, 55].

3.5 Promotion of early oral intake

One of the key objectives in the post-operative period for normally fed patients is the restoration of normal Gastro Intestinal (GI) function that allows an adequate food intake and a rapid recovery. A recent meta-analysis of controlled trials about early enteral or oral feeding versus 'nil by mouth' after major surgery showed no clear advantage in keeping patients fasting after elective surgery [56]. Early nourish reduced both the risk of any kind of infection and the mean hospitalisation. However, the risk of vomiting is increased in patients early fed and, in the absence of a multimodal anti-emetic therapy, early enteral feeding has been associated with intestinal swelling, impaired mobilisation and reduced pulmonary function [57]; for these reasons, it is essential to adopt a targeted strategy for post-operative nausea and vomiting (PONV).

The use of emetogenic drugs (neostigmine, opioids, certain gaseous anaesthetic agents, etc.) should be avoided, favouring agents that are less emetogenic. Patients at risk for PONV should receive prophylactic treatment (e.g. ondansetron, dexamethasone or droperidol) [58].

For malnourished patients, the use of oral nutritional supplements (ONS) in the post-operative period and for 8 weeks after discharge, demonstrated effective benefits in terms of recovery of nutritional status, protein balance and quality of life [47]. Positive effects on clinical outcomes from ONS have also been documented also in series of elective surgical patients who were not screened specifically for malnutrition [59]. The difference between these studies, which used traditional nutrition protocols, and ERAS programmes is that oral integration in the first started 4–5 days after surgery, in the second is commenced the day before surgery and continued for at least the first four post-operative days, in order to achieve recommended intakes of energy and protein [60, 61]. This point of ERAS programme is crucial also for patients undergoing minimally invasive thoracic surgery: in fact, we need not to forget the aim of 'a more quickly return to their baseline functional status' and we know from several authors that when used in combination, preoperative oral carbohydrate loading, epidural analgesia and early enteral nutrition, they improved the maintenance of nutritional status following surgery [25].

3.6 Early mobilisation and discharged criteria

Several factors are negatively influenced by bed rest: tissue oxygenation, pulmonary function, muscle strength, insulin resistance, muscle loss and risk of thromboembolism.

To minimise bed rest, the ERAS protocol should provide an organisation suitable for a plan of assistance with daily mobilisation targets and the patient should be nursed in an environment that stimulates mobilisation.

A useful stimulus can come, for example, from the compilation of a 'hospitalisation diary' in which the patient documents the activities performed on a daily basis; in this way, we can set more easily achievable goals such as, for example, that the patient remains out of bed at least 2 h on the day of surgery, increasing up to 6 h a day until discharge. As mentioned in the first part of the work, the ERAS project depends on the interaction of different professional figures: at this stage, the role of the nurse maintaining close and constant contact with the patient is crucial, and achieving decisive results also through the application of specific and innovative programmes such as 'nursing care map and programme'.

Patients can be discharged when they meet the following criteria:

- Good pain control with oral analgesia
- Taking solid food, no intravenous fluids
- Independently mobile or same level as prior to admission
- All of the above and willing to go home

The discharge process starts at the preadmission counselling session when it is determined if the patient lives alone and has any special needs (e.g. transport, social support, etc.). Problems that will delay discharge must be addressed at this time rather than once the patient has been admitted. Furthermore, it is crucial to set up a close follow-up on telephone monitoring of patient conditions followed by outpatient visits at predetermined times, the first of which generally falls to 15 and 30 days after discharge: to this, the key role played by a dedicated figure, the 'case manager', is of significant importance.

Author details

Domenico Viggiano[1*], Leonardo Politi[2], Alessandro Gonfiotti[2] and Andrea Droghetti[1]

1 Thoracic Surgery Unit, ASST, Mantova, Italy

2 Thoracic Surgery Unit, Careggi University Hospital, Florence, Italy

*Address all correspondence to: viggiano.md@gmail.com

References

[1] Fearon KC, Ljungqvist O, Von Meyenfeldt M, et al. Enhanced recovery after surgery: A consensus review of clinical care for patients undergoing colonic resection. Clinical Nutrition. 2005;**24**(3):466-477

[2] Weimann A, Braga M, Harsanyi L, et al. ESPEN guidelines on enteral nutrition: Surgery including organ transplantation. Clinical Nutrition. 2006;**25**:224-244

[3] Zhuang CL, Ye XZ, Zhang XD, Chen BC, Yu Z. Enhanced recovery after surgery programs versus traditional care for colorectal surgery: A meta-analysis of randomized controlled trials. Diseases of the Colon and Rectum. 2013;**56**(5):667-678

[4] Wind J, Polle SW, Fung Kon Jin PH, et al. Systematic review of enhanced recovery programmes in colonic surgery. The British Journal of Surgery. 2006;**93**:800-809

[5] Podore PC, Throop EB. Infrarenal aortic surgery with a 3-day hospital stay: A report on success with a clinical pathway. Journal of Vascular Surgery. 1999;**29**:787-792

[6] Gonfiotti A, Viggiano D, Droghetti A, et al. Enhanced recovery after surgery and video-assisted thoracic surgery lobectomy: The Italian VATS Group surgical protocol. Journal of Thoracic Disease. 2018;**10**(Suppl 4): S564-S570

[7] Gonfiotti A, Viggiano D, Bongiolatti S, et al. Enhanced recovery after surgery (ERAS®) in thoracic surgical oncology. Future Oncology. 2018;**14**(6s):33-40

[8] Willemsen PJ, Appeltans BM. Hospital stay of 2 days after open sigmoidectomy with a multimodal rehabilitation programme. British Journal of Surgery. 1999;**86**(7):968-969

[9] Koupparis A, Dunn J, Gillatt D, et al. Improvement of an enhanced recovery protocol for radical cystecomy. British Journal of Medical and Surgical Urology. 2010;**3**:237-240

[10] Eskicioglu C, Forbes SS, Aarts MA, Okrainec A, McLeod RS. Enhanced recovery after surgery (ERAS) programs for patients having colorectal surgery: A meta-analysis of randomized trials. Journal of Gastrointestinal Surgery. 2009;**13**:2321-2329

[11] Lassen K, Soop M, Nygren J, et al. Consensus review of optimal perioperative care in colorectal surgery: Enhanced recovery after surgery (ERAS) group recommendations. Archives of Surgery. 2009;**144**:961-969

[12] Kehlet H, Mogensen T. Hospital stay of 2 days after open sigmoidectomy with a multimodal rehabilitation programme. The British Journal of Surgery. 1999;**86**(2):227-230

[13] Kehlet H. Multimodal approach to control postoperative pathophysiology and rehabilitation. British Journal of Anaesthesia. 1997;**78**:606-617

[14] Ensor P. The functional silo syndrome. AME Target. 1988;**Spring**:16

[15] Egbert LD, Battit GE, Welch CE, Bartlett MK. Reduction of postoperative pain by encouragement and instruction of patients. A study of doctor–patient rapport. The New England Journal of Medicine. 1964;**270**:825-827

[16] Kiecolt-Glaser JK, Page GG, MacCallum RC, Glaser R. Psychological influences on surgical recovery. Perspectives from psychoneuroimmunology.

The American Psychologist. 1998;**53**(11):1209-1218

[17] Disbrow EA, Bennett HL, Owings JT. Effect of preoperative suggestion on postoperative gastrointestinal motility. The Western Journal of Medicine. 1993;**158**(5):488-492

[18] Ljungqvist O, Soreide E. Preoperative fasting. The British Journal of Surgery. 2003;**90**(4):400-406

[19] Eriksson LI, Sandin R. Fasting guidelines in different countries. Acta Anaesthesiologica Scandinavica. 1996;**40**(8 Part 2):971-974

[20] Soreide E, Fasting S, Raeder J. New preoperative fasting guidelines in Norway. Acta Anaesthesiologica Scandinavica. 1997;**41**(6):799

[21] Practice guidelines for preoperative fasting and the use of pharmacologic agents to reduce the risk of pulmonary aspiration: application to healthy patients undergoing elective procedures: A report by the American Society of Anesthesiologist Task Force on Preoperative Fasting. Anesthesiology. 1999;**90**(3):896-905

[22] Hausel J, Nygren J, Lagerkranser M, et al. A carbohydrate-rich drink reduces preoperative discomfort in elective surgery patients. Anesthesia and Analgesia. 2001;**93**(5):1344-1350

[23] Soop M, Nygren J, Myrenfors P, Thorell A, Ljungqvist O. Preoperative oral carbohydrate treatment attenuates immediate postoperative insulin resistance. American Journal of Physiology. Endocrinology and Metabolism. 2001;**280**(4):E576-E583

[24] Yuill KA, Richardson RA, Davidson HI, Garden OJ, Parks RW. The administration of an oral carbohydrate-containing fluid prior to major elective upper-gastrointestinal surgery preserves skeletal muscle mass postoperatievely—A randomised clinical trial. Clinical Nutrition. 2005;**24**(1):32-37

[25] Soop M, Carlson GL, Hopkinson J, et al. Randomized clinical trial of the effects of immediate enteral nutrition on metabolic responses to major colorectal surgery in an enhanced recovery protocol. The British Journal of Surgery. 2004;**91**(9):1138-1145

[26] British National Formulary. Oxford, UK: Pharmaceutical Press; 2003

[27] Uchida I, Asoh T, Shirasaka C, Tsuji H. Effect of epidural analgesia on postoperative insulin resistance as evaluated by insulin clamp technique. The British Journal of Surgery. 1988;**75**(6):557-562

[28] Scimia P, Basso Ricci E, Droghetti A, Fusco P. The ultrasound-guided continuous erector spinae plane block for postoperative analgesia in video-assisted thoracoscopic lobectomy. Regional Anesthesia and Pain Medicine. 2017;**42**(4):537

[29] Rigg JR, Jamrozik K, Myles PS, et al. Epidural anaesthesia and analgesia and outcome of major surgery: A randomised trial. Lancet. 2002;**359**(9314):1276-1282

[30] Holte K, Kehlet H. Epidural anaesthesia and analgesia—Effects on surgical stress responses and implications for postoperative nutrition. Clinical Nutrition. 2002;**21**(3):199-206

[31] Liu SS, Carpenter RL, Mackey DC, et al. Effects of perioperative analgesic technique on rate of recovery after colon surgery. Anesthesiology. 1995;**83**(4):757-765

[32] Niemi G, Breivik H. Adrenaline markedly improves thoracic epidural

analgesia produced by a low-dose infusion of bupivacaine, fentanyl and adrenaline after major surgery. A randomised, double-blind, cross-over study with and without adrenaline. Acta Anaesthesiologica Scandinavica. 1998;**42**(8):897-909

[33] Niemi G, Breivik H. Epinephrine markedly improves thoracic epidural analgesia produced by a small-dose infusion of ropivacaine, fentanyl, and epinephrine after major thoracic or abdominal surgery: A randomized, double-blinded crossover study with and without epinephrine. Anesthesia and Analgesia. 2002;**94**(6):1598-1605

[34] Niemi G, Breivik H. The minimally effective concentration of adrenaline in a low-concentration thoracic epidural analgesic infusion of bupivacaine, fentanyl and adrenaline after major surgery. A randomized, double-blind, dose-finding study. Acta Anaesthesiologica Scandinavica. 2003;**47**(4):439-450

[35] Jorgensen H, Wetterslev J, Moiniche S, Dahl JB. Epidural local anaesthetics versus opioid-based analgesic regimens on postoperative gastrointestinal paralysis, PONV and pain after abdominal surgery. Cochrane Database of Systematic Reviews. 2000;**4**:CD001893

[36] Ballantyne JC, Carr DB, deFerranti S, et al. The comparative effects of postoperative analgesic therapies on pulmonary outcome: Cumulative meta-analyses of randomized, controlled trials. Anesthesia and Analgesia. 1998;**86**(3):598-612

[37] Power I, Barratt S. Analgesic agents for the postoperative period. Nonopioids. Surgical Clinics of North America. 1999;**79**(2):275-295

[38] Kehlet H, Holte K. Effect of postoperative analgesia on surgical outcome. British Journal of Anaesthesia. 2001;**87**(1):62-72

[39] Das-Neves-Pereira JC, Bagan P, Coimbra-Israel AP, et al. Fast-track rehabilitation for lung cancer lobectomy: A five-year experience. European Journal of Cardio-Thoracic Surgery. 2009;**36**(2):383-391

[40] McKenna RJ Jr, Houck W, Fuller CB. Video-assisted thoracic surgery lobectomy: Experience with 1,100 cases. The Annals of Thoracic Surgery. 2006;**81**(2):421-425

[41] Harris CG, James RS, Tian DH, et al. Systematic review and meta-analysis of uniportal versus multiportal video-assisted thoracoscopic lobectomy for lung cancer. Annals of Cardiothoracic Surgery. 2016;**5**(2):76-84

[42] Jutley RS, Khalil MW, Rocco G. Uniportal vs standard three-port VATS technique for spontaneous pneumothorax: Comparison of post-operative pain and residual paraesthesia. European Journal of Cardio-Thoracic Surgery. 2005;**28**(1):43-46

[43] Gonfiotti A, Jaus MO, Viggiano D, et al. Uniportal videothoracoscopic surgery: Our indications and limits. Innovations (Phila). 2015;**10**(5):309-313

[44] Tamura M, Shimizu Y, Hashizume Y. Pain following thoracoscopic surgery: Retrospective analysis between single-incision and three-port video-assisted thoracoscopic surgery. Journal of Cardiothoracic Surgery. 2013;**8**:153

[45] Crisci R, Droghetti A, Migliore M, et al. Video-assisted thoracic lobectomy for lung cancer in Italy: The 'VATS Group' Project. Future Oncology. 2016;**12**:9-11

[46] Singhal S, Ferraris VA, Bridges CR, et al. Management of

alveolar air leaks after pulmonary resection. The Annals of Thoracic Surgery. 2010;**89**:1327-1335

[47] Brunelli A, Xiume F, Al Refai M, et al. Air leaks after lobectomy increase the risk of empyema but not of cardiopulmonary complications: A case-matched analysis. Chest. 2006;**130**:1150-1156

[48] Varela G, Jimenez MF, Novoa N, et al. Estimating hospital costs attributable to prolonged air leak in pulmonary lobectomy. European Journal of Cardio-Thoracic Surgery. 2005;**27**:329-333

[49] Temes RT, Willms CD, Endara SA, et al. Fissureless lobectomy. The Annals of Thoracic Surgery. 1998;**65**:282-284

[50] Dunning J, Prendergast B, Mackway-Jones K. Towards evidence-based medicine in cardiothoracic surgery: Best BETS. Interactive Cardiovascular and Thoracic Surgery. 2003;**2**:405-409

[51] Li S, Lv W, Zhou K, et al. Does the fissureless technique decrease the incidence of prolonged air leak after pulmonary lobectomy? Interactive Cardiovascular and Thoracic Surgery. 2017;**25**:122-124

[52] Nosotti M, Droghetti A, Luzzi L, et al. First Italian consensus conference on VATS lobectomy for NSCLC. Tumori. 2017;**103**:124-135

[53] Bjerregaard LS, Jensen K, Petersen RH, et al. Early chest tube removal after video-assisted thoracic surgery lobectomy with serous fluid production up to 500 ml/day. European Journal of Cardio-Thoracic Surgery. 2014;**45**:241-246

[54] Miyazaki T, Sakai T, Yamasaki N, et al. Chest tube insertion is one important factor leading to intercostal nerve impairment in thoracic surgery. General Thoracic and Cardiovascular Surgery. 2014;**62**:58-63

[55] Zhang X, Lv D, Li M, et al. The single chest tube versus double chest tube application after pulmonary lobectomy: A systematic review and meta-analysis. Journal of Cancer Research & Therapy. 2016;**12**:309-316

[56] Lewis SJ, Egger M, Sylvester PA, Thomas S. Early enteral feeding versus "nil by mouth" after gastrointestinal surgery: Systematic review and meta-analysis of controlled trials. British Medical Journal. 2001;**323**(7316):773-776

[57] Watters JM, Kirkpatrick SM, Norris SB, Shamji FM, Wells GA. Immediate postoperative enteral feeding results in impaired respiratory mechanics and decreased mobility. Annals of Surgery. 1997;**226**(3):369-377. Discussion 377-380

[58] Gan TJ, Meyer T, Apfel CC, et al. Consensus guidelines for managing postoperative nausea and vomiting. Anesthesia and Analgesia. 2003;**97**(1):62-71

[59] Beattie AH, Prach AT, Baxter JP, Pennington CR. A randomised controlled trial evaluating the use of enteral nutritional supplements postoperatively in malnourished surgical patients. Gut. 2000;**46**(6):813-818

[60] Smedley F, Bowling T, James M, et al. Randomized clinical trial of the effects of preoperative and postoperative oral nutritional supplements on clinical course and cost of care. The British Journal of Surgery. 2004;**91**(8):983-990

[61] Fearon KC, Luff R. The nutritional management of surgical patients: Enhanced recovery after surgery. The Proceedings of the Nutrition Society. 2003;**62**(4):807-811

Section 3

Surgery

Chapter 3

Single-Row Versus Double-Row Repair in Rotator Cuff Tears

Michael E. Hantes, Georgios I. Chalatsis and Georgios Mpakagiannis

Abstract

Rotator cuff (RC) tear is a common cause of shoulder pain and disability among adults. Surgical management of RC tears is recommended after conservative treatment failure. Due to the development of arthroscopic repair techniques, the use of the arthroscopic rotator cuff repair has become the gold standard. Single-row (SR) and double-row (DR) suture anchor repairs are the two most popular and commonly used arthroscopic techniques. However, the optimal arthroscopic surgical technique remains controversial in terms of clinical and biomechanical outcomes, healing, and re-tear rates. This chapter will focus on differences between these two techniques regarding biomechanics, clinical results, healing rate, and cost effectiveness.

Keywords: rotator, cuff, repair, single-row, double-row, versus, shoulder, arthroscopy

1. Introduction

The rotator cuff is a group of muscles and their tendons which is consisted by supraspinatus, infraspinatus, teres minor and subscapularis muscles (**Figures 1** and **2**). Rotator cuff tears can hinder the daily activities and the quality of life significantly in adult population. There is a high correlation between rotator cuff tears incidence and advancing age [1]. The overall prevalence of rotator cuff tears range from 20 to 30% for patients older than 60 years old and raises even more to 62%, in patients older than 80 years (regardless of symptoms), among the general population and in patients with a history of shoulder dislocation [1–4]. Partial thickness rotator cuff tears range from 15 to 32% in the general population and rises to 40% in dominant arm of asymptomatic elite overhead athletes [1]. The tear progression is correlated with the initial tear presentation. Patients with partial thickness rotator cuff tear can heal (10%) or become smaller (10%), but 53% progress and 28% become full-thickness tears [60]. On the other hand, patients with more than 50% initial tear had 55% chance the tear to progress [5]. Keener in his study of survivorship of asymptomatic degenerative rotator cuff tears, reported that full-thickness tears were 4.2 and 1.5 times more likely to enlarge than controls and partial tears respectively. Accordingly, tear progression was a risk factor for pain development and muscle degeneration [6]. Sex does not seem to play a significant role to the development of rotator cuff tears [6, 7], although there is a correlation between postmenopausal women, and an increase prevalence in asymptomatic rotator cuff tears [8]. Patients who have been operated in one shoulder for partial or full thickness

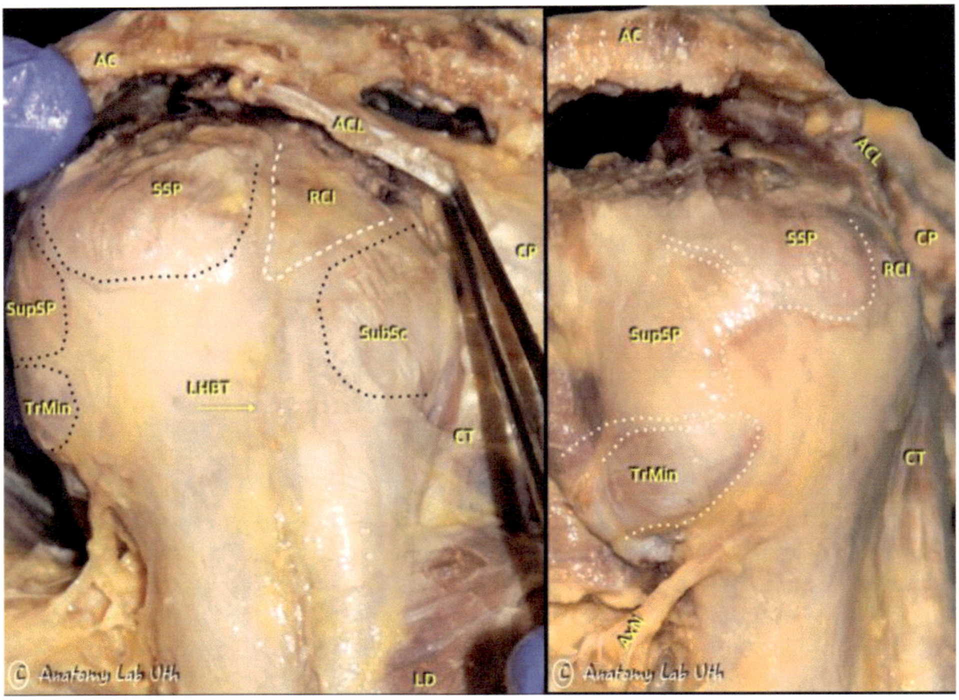

Figure 1.
*Frontal plane cross section of fresh frozen cadaveric shoulder specimen. SSPT, supraspinatus tendon; Arcap, articular capsule and the junction of the Arcap and SSPT is marked with the *; Rotcab, rotator cuff cable; RC, rotator cuff; TLHB, tendon of long head of humerus biceps; HH, humerus head (courtesy of A.H. Zibis Associate Professor of Anatomy, Department of Anatomy, Faculty of Medicine University of Thessaly).*

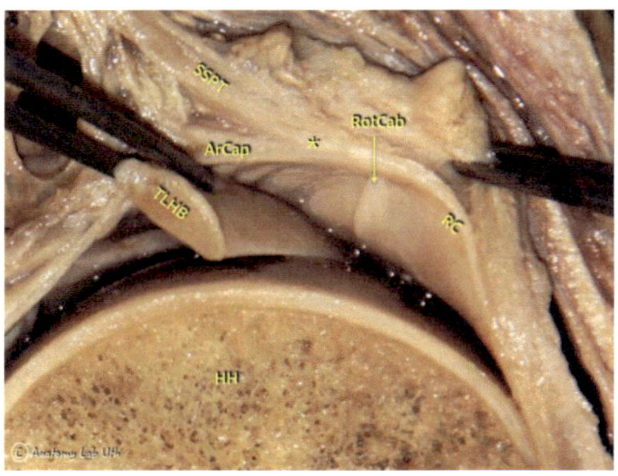

Figure 2.
Lateral and oblique posterolateral view of a fresh frozen cadaveric specimen of a right shoulder. AC, acromion; ACL, coracoacromial ligament; CP, coracoid process; TrMin, Teres Minor; SupSP, Infraspinatus; SSP, Supraspinatus; RCI, rotator cuff interval; SubSc, subscapularis; LD, latissimus dorsi; AxN, axillary nerve (courtesy of A.H. Zibis associate professor of anatomy, Department of Anatomy, Faculty of Medicine University of Thessaly).

tendon tear are in increased risk of developing the same on the opposite shoulder [9]. The possibility of a bilateral tear is nearly 50% in patients over 60 years old [1]. Other important predisposing factors are history of trauma, hypercholesterolemia, occupational demands [10], smoking [11], a positive family history [12] and the body posture with higher prevalence in individuals with kyphotic-lordotic, flat back and sway-back posture than people with ideal alignment [13, 14].

Grade	
I	<3 mm (<25% thickness)
II	3–6 mm (25–50%)
III	>6 mm (>50%)
Location	
A	Articular sided
B	Bursal sided
C	Intratendinous

Table 1.
Ellman's classification of partial thickness rotator cuff tars.

The classification of the rotator cuff tears is based on Ellman's classification of partial-thickness rotator cuff tears [15] and is categorized based on the grade of the tear and the location (**Table 1**). Snyder [16] classified the size of the defect by its superficial extension. Grade I tears represent a synovial irritation or capsular fraying in an area less than 1 cm, Grade II tear is a lesion with a fraying and failure of some rotator cuff fibers, and additionally synovial, bursal, or capsular injury in an area smaller than 2 cm. Grade III is a tear of the tendon fibers less than 3 cm. Fraying and fragmentation of the tendon and a tear more than 3 cm, involving more than a single tendon, is assessed as a grade IV lesion. Partial articular supraspinatus tendon avulsion, with a traumatic etiology is described as a special form of a type AIII or AIV.

The International Society of Arthroscopy, Knee Surgery and Ortopaedic Sports Medicine Shoulder Committee in its consensus recommendations for the RC tears classification system advices five important factors to be accounted: location, extension, pattern, fatty atrophy and retraction [17].

Adequate initial fixation plays a key role in achieving successful restoration of the rotator cuff tear. The primary function of the rotator cuff is to keep the head of the humerus centered into the glenoid fossa permitting a single center of rotation while enabling abduction or forward flexion [18, 19]. This is achieved with the balance of force couples around the glenohumeral joint. Two couple forces exist in the shoulder joint, the coronal force couple, with Deltoid versus inferior rotator cuff (Infraspinatus, Scapularis and Teres Minor) which opposes the force created by Deltoid muscle [20] and the transverse force couple [21, 22] which is a balance between Scapularis anteriorly and Infraspinatus and Teres Minor posteriorly. In massive RC tears, with the involvement of Infraspinatus muscle, along with Supraspinatus, the force couples are misbalancing, leading to posterosuperior migration of the head and incapability to maintain a steady fulcrum of motion.

Important anatomic factors for the success of the surgical reconstruction include the restoration of the footprint contact area, and the adequate compression of the tendon on it [23, 24], along with the rotator cuff muscles, tendon and bone quality [13]. Although various techniques like open and mini open surgery have been used in the past, the advance of arthroscopic repair techniques, with the development of the suture anchors, have become more and more popular [25]. Although there was no significant difference between re-tear rates, functional and pain scores, between mini-open and arthroscopic reconstruction, patients who received arthroscopic repair had fewer post-operation complications and returned earlier to work [18, 26]. However, there is still controversy which arthroscopic technique of the two most commonly used - single-row (SR) and the double-row (DR) – provide better clinical results [19].

2. Operative techniques

According to the geometric tear patterns of the rotator cuff, four different types of repairs have been described [28]. Type 1 is crescent-shaped tears, relatively short and wide. The medial to lateral length of these tears is less than anterior to posterior width and can be fixed directly to the bone bed on the greater humeral tuberosity [29–32]. Type II is longitudinal (U- and L-shaped) tears. The medial-to-lateral length of these tears is greater than the anterior-to-posterior width (**Figure 3**). These types of tears are usually repaired by a side to side convergence technique, reducing the strain of the lateral free margin of the cuff, with suture anchors, without tension [29, 31, 32]. Type III, are large contracted tears, long and wide. The tendon edge is too long and cannot be pulled directly to the bone and additionally too wide for the edges to be closed side to side. Interval slides or partial repairs are necessary for this type of lesions [30, 33–38]. Finally, type IV tears are related with significant glenohumeral arthritis and complete loss of the acromiohumeral interspace. These massive lesions are not repairable by arthroscopic or open surgery and the current treatment concept is arthroplasty.

The suture anchor techniques that are used more often are the single row (SR) and the double row (DR). Both of them have modifications. In the SR repair technique, there is the knotted and knotless repair, and in DR repair technique, there is the simple DR and the transosseous equivalent.

In the SR technique, two (or even more) double-loaded suture anchors are placed in a single row into the greater tuberosity at the lateral edge of the foot-print of the tendon's insertion (**Figures 4** and **5**). Anchor sutures are passed and tied in a simple or horizontal-mattress configuration, in a single anterior–posterior row in the knotted repair. The sutures are passed through the tendon, evenly spaced and 5 mm from the torn edge and then secured with knots and repair is achieved with a minimal tension. For the knotless repair the mattress suture are driven through the torn tendon with the help of an implant. A hole for the anchor is created into the corresponding position on the footprint. Both limbs of the suture are passing through the implant and the anchor and suture construct implanted together into the prepared hole. The anchor is reducing and locking the tendon to the bone [39] (**Figures 6–8**).

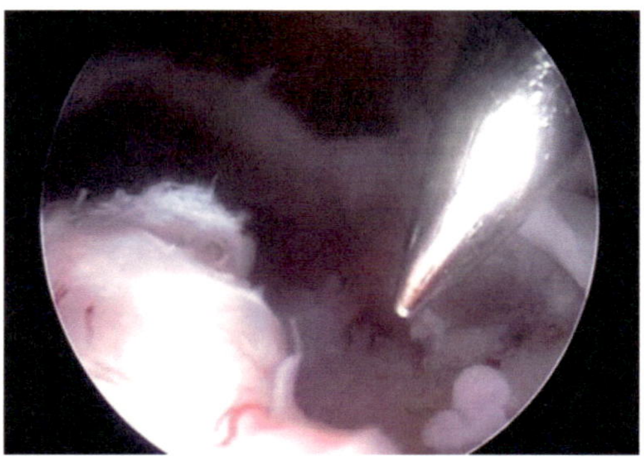

Figure 3.
Type II rotator cuff tear. Placement of guide for suture anchor.

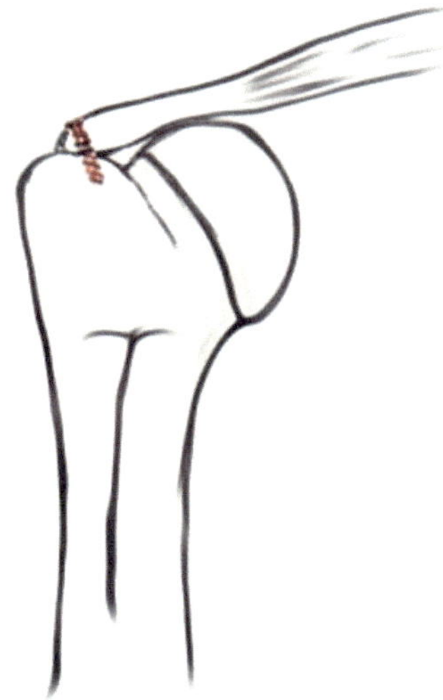

Figure 4.
Coronal view of Single Row suture anchors.

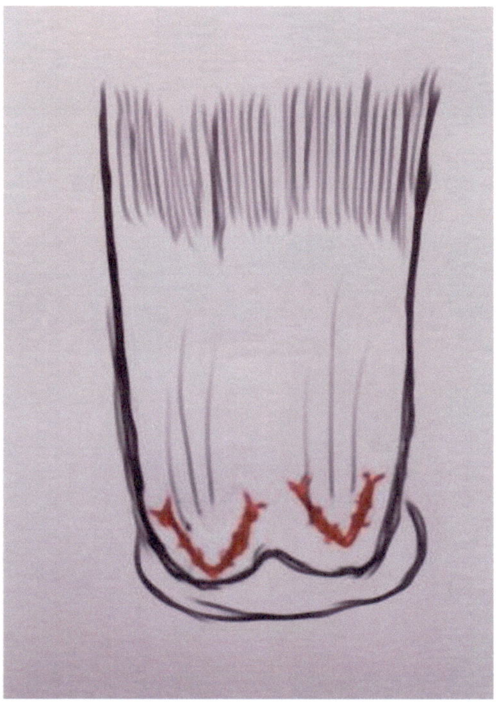

Figure 5.
Axial view of Single Row suture anchors.

In the DR repair technique two rows of anchors are placed, one medial, adjacent to the articular cartilage in the anatomical neck and the other lateral, in the greater tubercle, in order to provide better anatomical footprint restoration [40, 41] (**Figures 9** and **10**). In order for the repair structure not to lead to excessive tension,

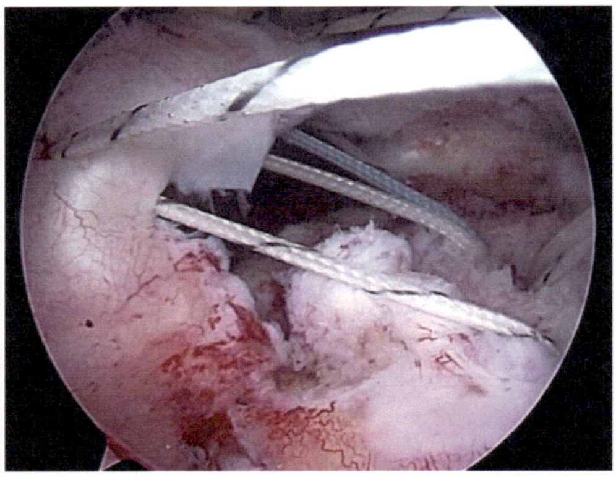

Figure 6.
Sutures through the tendon in a SR repair.

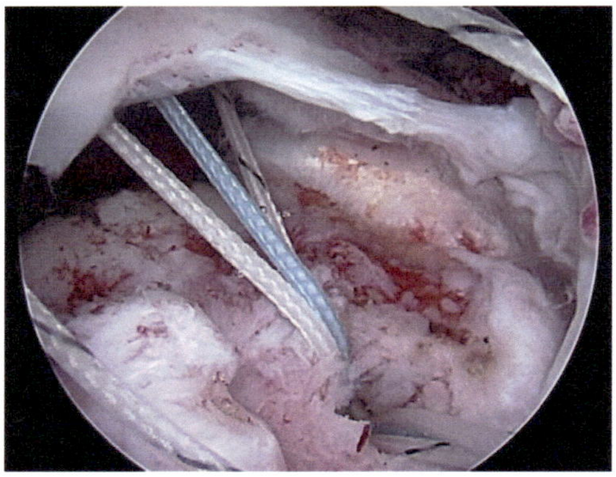

Figure 7.
A triple suture loaded anchor with sutures passed through the tendon in a SR repair.

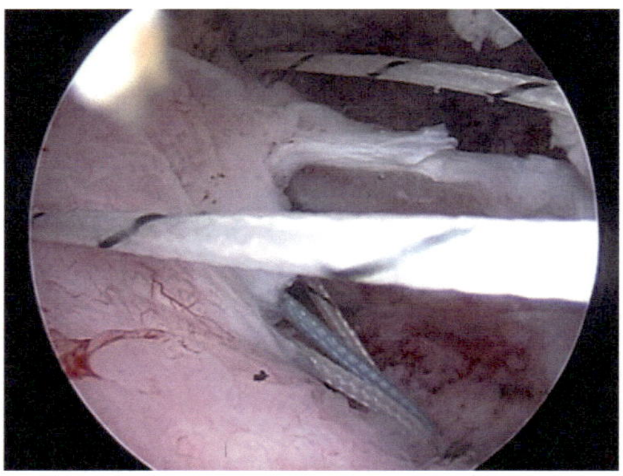

Figure 8.
All sutures anchors passed through the tendon.

the torn tendon should be mobilized to ensure that it can reach the lateral side of greater tubercle. Firstly, the medial row suture anchors are placed through at least 10–12 mm apart from each other and 12–15 mm medially from the lateral edge of the torn rotator cuff tendon in a horizontal mattress fashion [42]. Subsequently, the lateral row suture anchors are placed along the lateral side of greater tubercle. The lateral row suture anchors are passed through the lateral side of the tendon by simple suture configuration and tied in way that it will create a suture bridge construct.

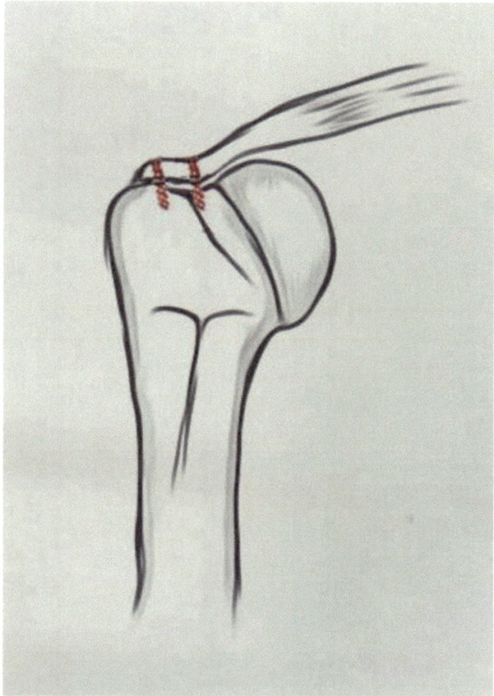

Figure 9.
Coronal view of Double Row suture anchors.

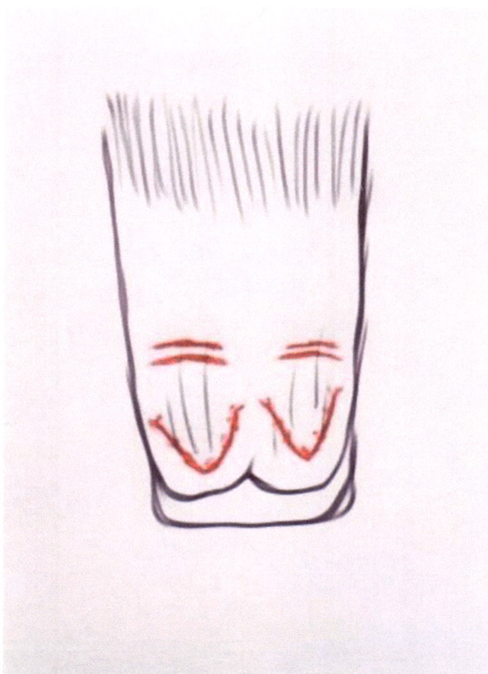

Figure 10.
Axial view of Double Row suture anchors.

After that, the medial row sutures are tied with proper tension. Depending on the size of the tear, the preference about the number of the anchors may vary. Throughout, the most important point is the assurance that remains adequate

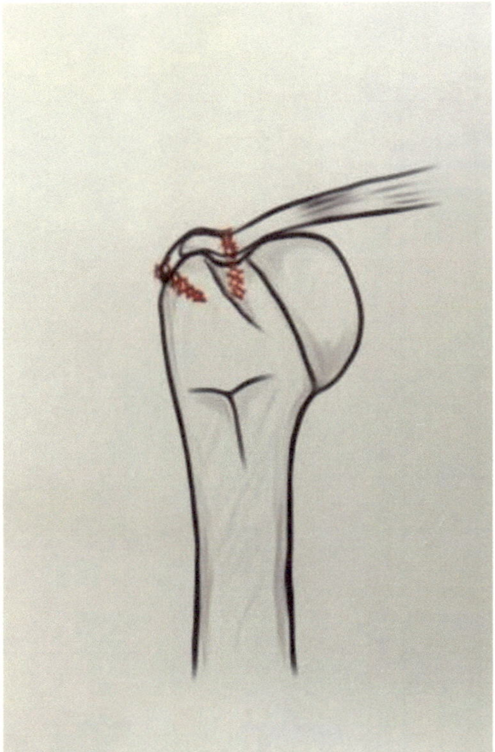

Figure 11.
Coronal view of Transosseous equivalent repair.

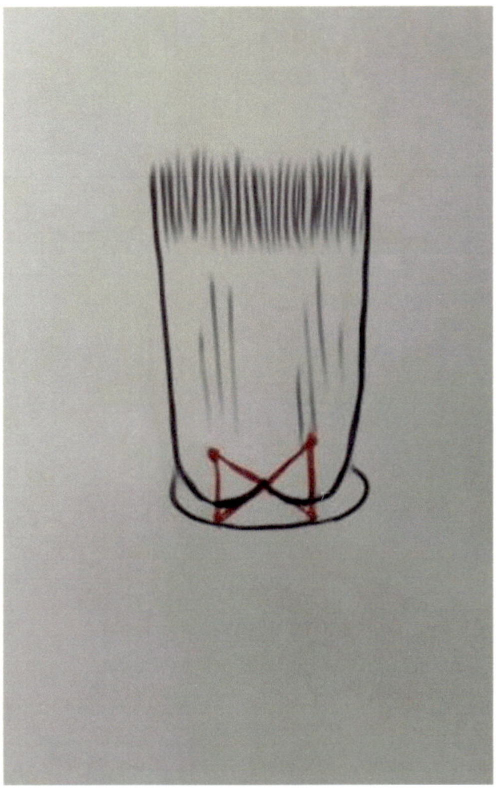

Figure 12.
Axial view of Transosseous equivalent repair.

block of bone between the anchors in order to prevent the risk of overcrowding and anchor failure.

Transosseous equivalent repair with knotless anchors is a modification of traditional double row technique. After the medial row sutures have been placed 12–15 mm medial to the torn edge, they are tied in a mattress fashion. Both limbs of each suture from the medial anchors are then crossed over and brought laterally down to the lateral aspect of greater tuberosity, compressing the tendon to the anatomical footprint. In this way, tissue strangulation by the knots is decreased and tendon vascularity is better preserved (**Figures 11** and **12**).

3. Biomechanics

Biomechanics analysis holds an important place in comparing those two techniques. A lot of cadaveric and animal model has been demonstrated over the times but none of them can foretell the healing potential but surely can answer about the failure strength (especially at day one) each technique provides, footprint restoration, gap formation and the pros and cons of each method. So, each technique must be biomechanically adequate in order to provide a good healing environment and provide adequate fixation until the healing is done.

The mandatory biomechanical features that should be provided are high initial fixation strength, minimal gap formation and the continuation of mechanical stability until the durable bone-tendon repair is completed [43]. In matter of biomechanics, DR repair seems to be far more superior to SR technique. Several studies have shown that DR has the capacity to restore the anatomical footprint almost to 100% something that it cannot be achieved while using SR repair technique and can lead to substantial morbidity. Also, it is shown that DR is a sturdier technique and can reduce the tendon-bone interface mobility and that can lead to better healing environment [44–46].

Although there are some data suggesting that there may be no difference in biomechanical features between those two techniques, most studies support that DR repair has a stronger structure in RC repair due to better restoration of the footprint, higher initial and failure strength, increased footprint contact pressure and lesser gap formation risk and all that can lead to better healing environment and enable more aggressive postoperative rehabilitation [47, 48].

4. Healing and re-tear rate

Healing of a torn rotator cuff is a formation of a continuous layer of tissue from the rotator cuff muscle to its insertion on the greater tuberosity [49]. The rotator cuff healing without surgical repair has been shown to be lower and inadequate in quality as demonstrated in animal models. A significant problem after RC repair is the re-tear on non-healing of the tendon [50, 51]. There are several factors that influence the re-tear rates such as age, preoperative tear size, degree of muscular atrophy, degree of fatty infiltration, surgical technique and inappropriate post-operative rehabilitation [52]. There are numerous studies in the literature that investigate the structural integrity and re-tear rates of these surgical techniques. The retrospective study of Sugaya et al. one of the longest follow up studies which compares the re-tear rates of SR and DR technique, they found 56% re-tear rate in patients treated with SR and 27% re-tear rate in patients who underwent DR repair after 3 years of follow up [53]. Several studies in the literature showed that patients who underwent RC repair and have re-rupture of the rotator cuff tendon are in better condition in terms of pain than they were pre-operative [54], but other studies directly contradict that and suggest that re-ruptures are associated with loss of strength [55]. Charousset et al. investigated re-tear rates of the patients using CT arthrography and demonstrated that anatomic healing was better in DR repair than SR [56]. The radiological outcomes of SR and DR repair in medium size rotator cuff tears using MR arthrography was examined by Tudisco et al. and detected a lower re-tear rate in DR technique [57]. A systematic review by Duquin et al. [58] also showed that in RC tears more than 10 mm in size, SR repair has significantly larger re-tear rates than DR repair, also in a meta-analysis which compared SR re-tear rates with DR rates revealed bigger re-tear rate in SR repair especially in partial thickness re-tears [27]. Finally, in patients who are in high risk of shoulder stiffness after the operation and are in need for accelerated rehabilitation protocol Franceschi et al. proved that DR repair had significant lower rates of re-tear than SR [59]. In a meta-analysis by Millet et al. in which they concluded only level of evidence I studies they found higher rates of re-tear in SR 25.9% compared to DR repair 14.2% [60]. Finally, a prospective comparative study by Hantes et al. [61] proved that double-row repair provides superior tendon healing compared to single-row and also DR must be considered in patients <55 years with medium to large RC tears.

However, RC healing has questionable association with outcomes. Tear and patient age, comorbidities, Nonsteroidal Anti-Inflammatory Drugs (NSAIDs), smoking status, osteoporosis and tendon shortening and retraction, affects negatively the outcomes. Surgical repair techniques and rehabilitation play important role but have varying degrees of impact on the final result [62–64].

The general consensus in the literature is because of the biomechanical superiorities od DR repair, which are demonstrated in experimental environments carry over healing capacity and lead to lower re-tear rates.

5. Cost

The DR technique has some obvious disadvantages such as time consuming, higher difficulty and it's more expensive. These factors are more significant if the final outcome is not associated with better clinical results than SR repair. In their study, Bisson et al. [65] tried to calculate the costs of the US healthcare system of transition from SR to DR rotator cuff repair and to calculate the decrease in re-operations for re-tear that DR rotator cuff repair would need to accomplish in order to render the transition cost-neutral. The calculated cost for SR repair technique was $7572 while for DR repair technique was $12,979. They concluded that DR repair would require a large decrease in revision surgery rates to justify this difference in cost.

Genuario et al. [66] in their study evaluated two different group of patients. One with >3 cm rotator cuff tear and another one with <3 cm and created a decision-analytic model to measure the cost-effect of DR repair compared to SR repair. It was found that DR rotator cuff repair was not cost-effective in any size of tear.

On the other hand, a later cost-utility analysis by Huang et al. [67], indicated that even though there were no significant differences in functional or quality-of-life measures between single row and double row repair technique, double row repair was more cost effective than SR. There was also noted that DR fixation was more economically friendly for tear larger than 3 cm.

According to all this and in conjunction to the absence of studies that correlate the cost of each repair technique with healing, re-tear rate, clinical outcomes and additional cost during follow up (failure of treatment, necessity for extra conservative treatment), there is no consensus with regards to the financial viability of one technique over the other one.

6. Functional and clinical outcomes

In both SR and DR techniques the functional shoulder scores, after rotator cuff repair, improve significantly. The clinical evaluation among several studies is based on many important aspects in patient's daily life, such as range of motion, function, strength, pain and general satisfaction. Some often-used scores are ASES (American Shoulder and Elbow Surgeons) shoulder scale [68], which is a subjective measurement that assess pain and level of function and it is scaled from 0 to 100, the Constant shoulder score [69], which combines subjective and objective data into a functional score on a scale also from 0 to 100, and the UCLA (University of California, Los Angeles) shoulder rating scale [70] that uses subjective and objective measurements that evaluate shoulder function on a scale of 0–35.

Several randomized controlled trials (RCTs) have been conducted comparing the two techniques. Many authors concluded that there is no statistically significant clinical difference between the two surgical methods. In 2009, Burks et al. [71] split evenly 40 patients in two repair groups (single versus double row) and evaluated their functional improvement without finding any difference. Aydin et al. [72] divided 64 patients evenly in two groups with a minimal 2 year follow up, with no significant difference in clinical outcome (Constant score) between them. Koh et al. [73] studied 62 patients (31 in each group) through clinical scores and patient satisfaction with no statistically important difference. Lapner et al. [74] did not find any significant difference in functional or quality of life outcomes in a heterogenous group of patients with tears of all sizes. Nicholas et al. [75] looking 49 patients in a prospective RCT found no differences between DR and SR repair for medium, large and massive rotator cuff tears in terms of outcome scores, clinical tests of shoulder function, shoulder range of movement (ROM) or shoulder strength.

Similar results were found also and in a systematic review and meta-analysis of 7 level I RCTs by Millet et al. [36], concluding that there were no detectable differences in improvement in outcomes scores (ASES, UCLA and Constant) between single row and double row repairs. The same result was found by Spiegl et al. [27], in a summary of eight meta-analysis comparing clinical differences between repairs for small and medium rotator cuff tears, in short and medium follow up.

On the other hand, Park et al. [77] whilst did not find significant functional difference in tears less than 3 cm, noted better results for the double row repair in tears larger than 3 cm. In a larger multicenter RCT by Carbonel et al. [78], with a minimum 2 year follow up and patients with large full thickness rotator cuff tears, DR repairs showed a significant difference in clinical outcomes (UCLA, Constant and ASES) compared with single row repair. A prospective RCT by Ma et al. [79] pointed that DR reconstruction showed better shoulder strength in patients with larger tear size (>3 cm) in comparison with SR.

In a more recent study, Hantes et al. [61] studied 66 individuals younger than 55 years old. Although there was no significant difference in outcomes scores observed between the two groups, they noted that patients in the DR group had a higher tendon healing rate ($p < 0.05$) and patients with healed tendon demonstrated superior clinical outcomes compared with patients who had retorn tendon ($p < 0.05$).

Saridakis et al. [80], despite the fact that in six studies found no significant differences, within their data, there was some evidence to support the use of DR repair in patients with large (>3 cm) tears.

Tasjian et al. [81] compared healing and function after single-row repair versus double row repair with a suture bridge technique for RC tears of size 1–3 cm and similar improvements in pain and function for a follow up period of 12 months.

In terms of re-tear rate, Franceschi [82] compared partial and full thickness re-tear after SR and DR rotator cuff repair. From the 52 patients equally distributed in two groups, there was no statistically significant difference neither in partial nor in full-thickness re-tears of RC. The same results have been observed by Carbonel et al. [78] and Barber [83] with no difference in both groups of partial or full thickness re-tear, no matter the technique. Park et al. [77] studied patients in groups according to the tear size also. They found lower re-tear rates with DR technique in large tears only. Koh et al. [73] in his RCT found no significant difference for full thickness re-tears in 6 out of 23 patients undergoing DR repair and 4 out of 24 patients undergoing SR repair. On the other hand, there was a significant difference for partial thickness re-tears with 1 patient out of 23 in DR group and 11 patients out of 24 in SR group. Franceschi et al. [59] detected a difference in overall re-tear rates in DR and SR repair groups but when examined each size of tear separately found no significant difference for partial and full thickness tears between the two groups.

In his recent meta-analysis, Sobhy et al. [84] noted that there was a statistically significant difference between groups only for partial thickness re-tears and not for full thickness re-tears. He also found that DR repair showed improved UCLA scores and a correlation between cuff integrity and functional outcomes. The authors also noted that long-term level III studies showed a direct correlation of both functional and cuff structural integrity, with DR repair technique being superior than SR. This seems to be in a contrast compared with previous studies [76, 85] which concluded that there is no correlation between cuff integrity and shoulder function. The reason probably is that they depended on short- or mid-term results which did not give enough time to the two repair techniques to demonstrate significant functional and structural results and also the sample size, the patient population and the inherent study to study variability.

Yang et al. [86] in their meta-analysis of the clinical effect of the rotator cuff repair in single and double row repairs in 29 studies noted that full-thickness re-tear had considerable effect on clinical outcome.

Despite the biomechanical privilege, footprint coverage and tendon-to-bone contact than could lead to better healing of DR and Suture bridge techniques [87–91], excessive contact pressure, that can lead to reduced blood flow to rotator cuff tendon [92], can be the reason for high rates of re-tear. Stress concentration around the medial anchors has been observed to lead to an increased risk of medial cuff failure [93–97]. Two types of tears have been described [95], type 1 is a failure at the tendon-bone interface and type 2 is medial cuff failure with remnant cuff attached to the greater tuberosity. Therefore, there is a necessity for technical modifications of the DR and Suture bridge techniques, minimizing the stress on medial anchors and decreasing the risk of medial strangulation and necrosis.

7. Conclusions

The increasing likelihood of occurrence RC tears with advancing age and longevity makes adequate RC repair a very challenging matter due to results in activity restriction and severe pain. Regarding the functional and clinical outcome, although there is no consensus between studies which repair technique is superior in general, it is well documented that studies with homogenous groups (regarding the size of the tear) indicate a slight superiority of the DR technique. The biomechanical evidence support the supremacy of the DR repair and the same result is applicable for re-rupture and healing rate, comparing with the SR technique. However, DR repair is more demanding for the surgeon technique. The learning curve is much higher than SR. Although that DR is a more expensive technique than SR, there is a necessity for more studies to be conducted to justify and correlate cost with healing, re-tear rate and clinical outcomes. Considering the existing evidence, the type of repair must be individualized according to the tear size. DR repair should be performed to patients with larger tears and in patients who are in need for accelerated rehabilitation, while patients with small tears can have the same clinical outcome with SR repair.

Acknowledgements

A.H. Zibis, Associate Professor of Anatomy, Department of Anatomy, Faculty of Medicine University of Thessaly.

Conflict of interest

The authors declare no conflict of interest.

Notes/thanks/other declarations

Special thanks to Christos Chalatsis for the drawings.

Abbreviations

RC	rotator cuff
SR	single row
DR	double row
SB	suture bridge
ROM	range of movement
RCT	randomized control trial
ASES	American shoulder and elbow surgeons
UCLA	University of California, Los Angeles
NSAIDs	nonsteroidal anti-inflammatory drugs

Author details

Michael E. Hantes*, Georgios I. Chalatsis and Georgios Mpakagiannis
Faculty of Medicine, Department of Orthopaedic Surgery, School of Health Sciences, University of Thessaly, Larisa, Greece

*Address all correspondence to: hantesmi@otenet.gr

References

[1] Yamaguchi K, Ditsios K, Middleton WD, Hildebolt CF, Galatz LM, Teefey SA. The demographic and morphological features of rotator cuff disease. A comparison of asymptomatic and symptomatic shoulders. The Journal of Bone and Joint Surgery. American Volume. 2006;**88**:1699-1704. PMID: 16882890

[2] Teunis T, Lubberts B, Reilly BT, Ring D. A systematic review and pooled analysis of the prevalence of rotator cuff disease with increasing age. Journal of Shoulder and Elbow Surgery. 2014;**23**:1913-1921. PMID: 25441568

[3] Fehringer EV, Sun J, VanOeveren LS, Keller BK, Matsen FA. Full-thickness rotator cuff tear prevalence and correlation with function and co-morbidities in patients sixty-five years and older. Journal of Shoulder and Elbow Surgery. 2008;**17**:881-885

[4] Moosmayer S, Smith HJ, Tariq R, Larmo A. Prevalence and characteristics of asymptomatic tears of the rotator cuff: An ultrasonographic and clinical study. Journal of Bone and Joint Surgery. British Volume (London). 2009;**91**:196-200

[5] Mall NA, Kim HM, Keener JD, et al. Symptomatic progression of asymptomatic rotator cuff tears: A prospective study of clinical and sonographic variables. The Journal of Bone and Joint Surgery. 2010;**92**(16):2623-2633

[6] Keener JD, Galatz LM, Teefey SA, et al. A prospective evaluation of survivorship of asymptomatic degenerative rotator cuff tears. The Journal of Bone and Joint Surgery. 2015;**97**(2):89-98. DOI: 10.2106/JBJS.N.00099. PMID: 25609434

[7] Pauly S, Stahnke K, Klatte-Schulz F, Wildemann B, Scheibel M, Greiner S. Do patient age and sex influence tendon cell biology and clinical/radiographic outcomes after rotator cuff repair? The American Journal of Sports Medicine. 2015;**43**:549-556

[8] Milgrom C, Schaffler M, Gilbert S, van Holsbeeck M. Rotator-cuff changes in asymptomatic adults. The effect of age, hand dominance and gender. Journal of Bone and Joint Surgery. British Volume (London). 1995;**77**:296-298

[9] Abate M, Schiavone C, Di Carlo L, Salini V. Prevalence of and risk factors for asymptomatic rotator cuff tears in postmenopausal women. Menopause. 2014;**21**:275-280

[10] Liem D, Buschmann VE, Schmidt C, Gosheger G, Vogler T, Schulte TL, et al. The prevalence of rotator cuff tears: Is the contralateral shoulder at risk? The American Journal of Sports Medicine. 2014;**42**:826-830

[11] Yamamoto A, Takagishi K, Osawa T, Yanagawa T, Nakajima D, Shitara H, et al. Prevalence and risk factors of a rotator cuff tear in the general population. Journal of Shoulder and Elbow Surgery. 2010;**19**:116-120

[12] Kim KC, Shin HD, Cha SM, Park JY. Repair integrity and functional outcome after arthroscopic conversion to a full-thickness rotator cuff tear: Articular- versus bursal-side partial tears. The American Journal of Sports Medicine. 2014;**42**:451-456

[13] Lee TQ. Current biomechanical concepts for rotator cuff repair. Clinics in Orthopedic Surgery. 2013;**5**(2):89-97

[14] Lindley K, Jones GL. Outcomes of arthroscopic versus open rotator cuff repair: A systematic review of the literature. American Journal of Orthopedics (Belle Mead, N.J.). 2010;**39**:592-600

[15] Ellman H. Diagnosis and treatment of incomplete rotator cuff tears. Clinical Orthopaedics and Related Research. 1 May 1990;(254):64-74

[16] Snyder SJ. Arthroscopic classification of rotator cuff lesions and surgical decision making. In: Shoulder Arthroscopy. 2nd ed. Philadelphia: Lippincott Williams & Wilkins; 2003. pp. 201-207

[17] Arce G, Bak K, Bain G, et al. Management of disorders of the rotator cuff: Proceedings of the ISAKOS Upper Extremity Committee Consensus Meeting. Arthroscopy. 2013;**29**:1840-1850

[18] Saha AK. Dynamic stability of the glenohumeral joint. Acta Orthopaedica Scandinavica. 1972;**42**:476-483

[19] Basmajian JV, Bazant FJ. Factors preventing downward dislocation of the adducted shoulder joint. An electromyographic and morphological study. The Journal of Bone and Joint Surgery. 1959;**41A**:1182-1186

[20] Inman VT, Saunders JB, Abbott LC. Observations of the function of the shoulder joint. 1944. Clinical Orthopaedics and Related Research. Sept 1996;(330):3-12

[21] Burkhart SS. Partial repair of massive rotator cuff tears: The evolution of a concept. The Orthopedic Clinics of North America. 1997;**28**:125-132

[22] Burkhart SS. A stepwise approach to arthroscopic rotator cuff repair based on biomechanical principles. Arthroscopy. 2000;**16**:82-90

[23] Roth KM, Warth RJ, Lee JT, Millett PJ, ElAttrache NS. Arthroscopic single-row versus double-row repair for full thickness posterosuperior rotator cuff tears: A critical analysis review. JBJS Reviews. 22 Jul 2014;**2**(7). DOI: 10.2106/JBJS.RVW.M.00081

[24] Park MC, Cadet ER, Levine WN, Bigliani LU, Ahmad CS. Tendon-to-bone pressure distributions at a repaired rotator cuff footprint using transosseous suture and suture anchor fixation techniques. The American Journal of Sports Medicine. 2005;**33**(8):1154-1159

[25] Colvin AC, Egorova N, Harrison AK, Moskowitz A, Flatow EL. National trends in rotator cuff repair. The Journal of Bone and Joint Surgery. American Volume. 2012;**94**(3):227-233

[26] Agrawal V, Stinson M. Ability and length of time to return to work after RCR in workers' compensation patient. Indiana Orthopaedic Journal. 2008;**2**:49

[27] Spiegl UJ, Euler SA, Millett PJ, Hepp P. Summary of meta-analyses dealing with single-row double-row repair techniques for rotator cuff tears. The Open Orthopaedics Journal. 2016;**10**(Suppl 1):330-338. DOI: 10.2174/1874325001610010330

[28] Davidson J, Burkhart SS. The geometric classification of rotator cuff tears: A system linking tear pattern to treatment and prognosis. Arthroscopy. 2010;**26**(3):417-424

[29] Burkhart SS, Danaceau SM, Pearce CE. Arthroscopic rotator cuff repair: Analysis of results by tear size and by repair technique-margin convergence versus direct tendon-to-bone repair. Arthroscopy. 2001;**17**:905-912

[30] Davidson JF, Burkhart SS, Richards DP, Campbell SE. Use of preoperative magnetic resonance imaging to predict rotator cuff tear pattern and method of repair. Arthroscopy. 2005;**21**:1428.e1-1428.e10

[31] Burkhart SS. Current concepts: A stepwise approach to arthroscopic rotator cuff repair based on biomechanical principles. Arthroscopy. 2000;**16**:82-90

[32] Lo IK, Burkhart SS. Biomechanical principles of arthroscopic repair of the rotator cuff. Operative Techniques in Orthopaedics. 2002;**12**:140-155

[33] Lo IK, Burkhart SS. Arthroscopic repair of massive, contracted, immobile rotator cuff tears using single and double interval slides: Technique and preliminary results. Arthroscopy. 2004;**20**:22-33

[34] Burkhart SS, Nottage WM, Ogilvie-Harris DJ, Kohn HS, Pachelli A. Partial repair of irreparable rotator cuff tears. Arthroscopy. 1994;**10**:363-370

[35] Tauro JC. Arthroscopic rotator cuff repair: Analysis of technique and results at 2- and 3-year follow-up. Arthroscopy. 1998;**14**:45-51

[36] Tauro JC. Arthroscopic "interval slide" in the repair of large rotator cuff tears. Arthroscopy. 1999;**15**:527-530

[37] Cordasco FA, Bigliani LU. The rotator cuff: Large and massive tears. Techniques of open repair. Orthopedic Clinics of North America. 1997;**28**:179-193

[38] Codd TP, Flatow EL. Anterior acromioplasty, tendon mobilization and direct repair of massive rotator cuff tears. In: Burkhead WZ, editor. Rotator Cuff Disorders. Vol. 330. Baltimore: Williams & Wilkins; 1996

[39] Gartsman GM, Hammerman SM. Full-thickness tears: Arthroscopic repair. The Orthopedic Clinics of North America. 1997;**28**:83-98

[40] Lo KYI, Burkhart SS. Double-row arthroscopic rotator cuff repair: Re-establishing the footprint of the rotator cuff. Arthroscopy. 2003;**19**(9):1035-1042

[41] Snyder SJ. Shoulder Arthroscopy. 2nd ed. Philadelphia: Lippincott Williams & Wilkins; 2002

[42] AydinN KB, Gurcan M, Ozsahin MK. Arthroscopic double-row rotator cuff repair: A comprehensive review of the literature. SICOT Journal;**4**:57. DOI: 10.1051/sicotj/2018048

[43] Gerber C, Schneeberger AG, Perren SM, Nyffeler RW. Experimental rotator cuff repair. A preliminary study. The Journal of Bone and Joint Surgery. 1999;**81**:1281-1290

[44] Brady PC, Arrigoni P, Burkhart SS. Evaluation of residual rotator cuff defects after ın vivo single- versus double-row rotator cuff repairs. Arthroscopy. 2006;**22**:1070-1075

[45] Meier SW, Meier JD. Rotator cuff repair: The effect of double-row fixation on three-dimensional repair site. Journal of Shoulder and Elbow Surgery. 2006;**15**:691-696

[46] Milano G, Grasso A, Zarelli D, et al. Comparison between single-row and double-row rotator cuff repair: A biomechanical study. The Knee Surgery, Sports Traumatology, Arthroscopy. Jan 2008;**16**(1):75-80. DOI: 10.1007/s00167-007-0382-0. [Epub 8 Aug 2007]

[47] Mahar A, Tamborlane J, Oka R, et al. Single-row suture anchor repair of the rotator cuff is biomechanically equivalent to double-row repair in a bovine model. Arthroscopy. 2007;**23**:1265-1270

[48] Nelson CO, Sileo MJ, Grossman MG, Serra-Hsu F. Single-row modified mason-allen versus double-row arthroscopic rotator cuff repair: A biomechanical and surface area comparison. Arthroscopy. 2008;**24**:941-948

[49] Mall NA, Tanaka MJ, Choi LS, Paletta GA. Factors affecting rotator cuff healing. The Journal of Bone and Joint Surgery. American Volume. 2014;**96**:778-788. DOI: 10.2106/JBJS.M.00583

[50] Harryman DT, Mack LA, Wang KY, Jackins SE, Richardson ML, Matsen FA. Repairs of the rotator cuff. Correlation of functional results with integrity of the cuff. Journal of Bone and Joint Surgery. 1991;**73**(7):982-989. DOI: 10.2106/00004623-199173070-00004

[51] Lafosse L, Brzoska R, Toussaint B, Gobezie R. The outcome and structural integrity of arthroscopic rotator cuff repair with use of the double-row suture anchor technique. Surgical technique. The Journal of Bone and Joint Surgery. 2008;**90**(Suppl 2 Pt 2):275-286. DOI: 10.2106/JBJS.H.00388

[52] Galanopoulos I, Ilias A, Karliaftis K, Papadopoulos D, Ashwood N. The impact of re-tear on the clinical outcome after rotator cuff repair using open or arthroscopic techniques: A systematic review. The Open Orthopaedics Journal. 2017;**11**(Suppl 1):95-107. DOI: 10.2174/1874325001711010095.M4

[53] Sugaya H, Maeda K, Matsuki K, Moriishi J. Repair integrity and functional outcome after arthroscopic double row rotator cuff repair: A prospective outcome study. The Journal of Bone and Joint Surgery. 2007;**89**:953-960

[54] Galatz LM, Ball CM, Teefey SA, Middleton WD, Yamaguchi K. The outcome and repair integrity of completely arthroscopically repaired large and massive rotator cuff tears. The Journal of Bone and Joint Surgery. American Volume. 2004;**86-A**(2):219-224

[55] Boileau P, Brassart N, Watkinson DJ, Carles M, Hatzidakis AM, Krishnan SG. Arthroscopic repair of full-thickness tears of the supraspinatus: Does the tendon really heal? The Journal of Bone and Joint Surgery. American Volume. 2005;**87**(6):1229-1240. DOI: 10.2106/JBJS.D.02035

[56] Charousset C, Grimberg J, Duranthon LD. The time for functional recovery after arthroscopic rotator cuff repair: Correlation with tendon healing controlled by computed tomography arthrography. Arthroscopy. 2008;**24**:25-33

[57] Tudisco C, Bisicchia S, Savarese E. Single-row vs double-row arthroscopic rotator cuff repair: Clinical and 3 Tesla MR arthrography results. BMC Musculoskeletal Disorders. 2013;**14**:43

[58] Duquin TR, Buyea C, Bisson LJ. Which method of rotator cuff repair leads to thehighest rate of structural healing? A systematic review. The American Journal of Sports Medicine. 2010;**38**(4):835-841. DOI: 10.1177/0363546509359679

[59] Franceschi F, Papalia R, Franceschetti E, et al. Double-row repair lowers the re-tear risk after accelerated rehabilitation, double-row repair lowers the re-tear risk after accelerated rehabilitation. American Journal of Sports Medicine. 2016;**44**(4):948-956. DOI: 10.1177/0363546515623031

[60] Millett PJ, Warth RJ, Dornan GJ. Clinical and structural outcomes after arthroscopic single-row versus double-row rotator cuff repair: A systematic review and meta-analysis of level I randomized clinical trials. Journal of Shoulder and Elbow Surgery. 2014;**23**:586-597

[61] Hantes ME, Ono Y, Raoulis VA, Doxariotis N, Venouzioy A, Zibis A, et al. Arthroscopic single-row versus double-row suture bridge technique for rotator cuff tears in patients younger than 55 years: A prospective comparative study. The American Journal of Sports Medicine. 2018;**46**(1):116-121. DOI: 10.1177/0363546517728718

[62] Cho NS, Rhee YG. The factors affecting the clinical outcome and

integrity of arthroscopically repaired rotator cuff tears of the shoulder. Clinics in Orthopedic Surgery. 2009;**1**:96-104. DOI: 10.4055/cios.2009.1.2.96

[63] Abtahi AM, Granger EK, Tashjian RZ. Factors affecting healing after arthroscopic rotator cuff repair. World Journal of Orthopedics. 2015;**6**:211-220. DOI: 10.5312/wjo.v6.i2.211

[64] Chung SW, Oh JH, Gong HS, Kim JY, Kim SH. Factors affecting rotator cuff healing after arthroscopic repair: Osteoporosis as one of the independent risk factors. The American Journal of Sports Medicine. 2011;**39**:2099-2107. DOI: 10.1177/0363546511415659

[65] Bisson L, Zivaljevic N, Sanders S. A cost analysis of single-row versus double-row and suture bridge rotator cuff repair methods. Knee Surgery Sports Traumatology, Arthroscopy. 2015;**23**:487-493. DOI: 10.1007/s00167-012-2338-2

[66] Genuario JW, Donegan RP, Hamman D. The cost-effectiveness of single-row compared with double-row arthroscopic rotator cuff repair. The Journal of Bone and Joint Surgery. 2012;**94**(15):1369-1377. DOI: 10.2106/JBJS.J.01876

[67] Huang AL, Thavorn K, van Katwyk S, MacDonald P, Lapner P. Double-row arthroscopic rotator cuff repair is more cost-effective than single-row repair. Journal of Bone and Joint Surgery. 2017;**99**(20):1730-1736. DOI: 10.2106/JBJS.16. 01044

[68] Richards RR, An KN, Bigliani LU, et al. A standardized method for the assessment of shoulder function. Journal of Shoulder and Elbow Surgery. 1994;**3**:347-352

[69] Apreleva M, Ozbaydar M, Fitzgibbons PG, Warner JJ. Rotator cuff tears: The effect of the reconstruction method on three-dimensional repair site area. Arthroscopy. 2002;**18**:519-526

[70] Ellman H, Hanker G, Bayer M. Repair of the rotator cuff: End-result study of factors influencing reconstruction. The Journal of Bone and Joint Surgery. American Volume. 1986;**68**:1136-1144

[71] Burks RT, Crim J, Brown N, Fink B, Greis PE. A prospective randomized clinical trial comparing arthroscopic single- and double-row rotator cuff repair: Magnetic resonance imaging and early clinical evaluation. The American Journal of Sports Medicine. 2009;**37**:674-682

[72] Aydin N, Kocaoglu B, Guven O. Single-row versus double-row arthroscopic rotator cuff repair in small- to medium-sized tears. Journal of Shoulder and Elbow Surgery. 2010;**19**(5):722-725. DOI: 10.1016/j.jse.2009.11.053

[73] Koh KH, Kang KC, Lim TK, Shon MS, Yoo JC. Prospective randomized clinical trial of single- versus double-row suture anchor repair in 2- to 4-cm rotator cuff tears: Clinical and magnetic resonance imaging results. Arthroscopy. 2011;**27**:453-462

[74] Lapner PLC, Sabri E, Rakhra K, et al. A multicenter randomized controlled trial comparing single-row with double-row fixation in arthroscopic rotator cuff repair. The Journal of Bone and Joint Surgery. American Volume. 2012;**94**(14): 1249-1257. DOI: 10.2106/JBJS.K.00999

[75] Nicholas SJ, Lee SJ, Mullaney MJ, et al. Functional outcomes after double-row versus single-row rotator cuff repair: A prospective randomized trial. Orthopaedic Journal of Sports Medicine. 2016;**4**(10). DOI: 10.1177/2325967116667398

[76] Millett PJ, Warth RJ, Dornan GJ, Lee JT, Spiegl UJ. Clinical and structural outcomes after arthroscopic single-row versus double-row rotator cuff repair: A systematic review and meta-analysis of level I randomized clinical trials. The Journal of Shoulder and Elbow Surgery. 2014;**23**(4):586-597. DOI: 10.1016/j.jse.2013.10.006

[77] Park JY, Lhee SH, Choi JH, Park HK, Yu JW, Seo JB. Comparison of the clinical outcomes of single- and double-row repairs in rotator cuff tears. The American Journal of Sports Medicine. 2008;**36**:1310-1316

[78] Carbonel I, Martinez AA, Calvo A, Ripalda J, Herrera A. Single-row versus double-row arthroscopic repair in the treatment of rotator cuff tears: A prospective randomized clinical study. International Orthopaedics. 2012;**36**(9):1877-1883. DOI: 10.1007/s00264-012-1559-9

[79] Ma H-L, Chiang E-R, H-TH W, et al. Clinical outcome and imaging of arthroscopic single-row and double-row rotator cuff repair: A prospective randomized trial. Arthroscopy. 2012;**28**(1):16-24. DOI: 10.1016/j.arthro.2011.07.003

[80] Saridakis P, Jones G. Outcomes of single-row and double-row arthroscopic rotator cuff repair: A systematic review. The Journal of Bone and Joint Surgery. American Volume. 2010;**92**(3):732-742. DOI: 10.2106/JBJS.I.01295

[81] Tashjian RZ, Granger EK, Chalmers PN. Healing rates and functional outcomes after triple-loaded single-row versus transosseous-equivalent double-row rotator cuff tendon repair. Orthopaedic Journal of Sports Medicine. 2018;**6**(11):2325967118805365

[82] Franceschi F, Ruzzini L, Longo UG, Martina FM, Zobel BB, Maffulli N, et al. Equivalent clinical results of arthroscopic single-row and double-row suture anchor repair for rotator cuff tears: A randomized controlled trial. American Journal of Sports Medicine. 2007;**35**(8):1254-1260. DOI: 10.1177/0363546507302218

[83] Barber FA. Triple-loaded single-row versus suture-bridge double-row rotator cuff tendon repair with platelet-rich plasma fibrin membrane: A randomized controlled trial. Orthopaedic Journal of Sports Medicine. 2016;**32**(5):753-761. DOI: 10.1016/j.arthro.2015.11.020

[84] Sobhy MH, Khater AH, Hassan MR, El Shazly O. Do functional outcomes and cuff integrity correlate after single- versus double-row rotator cuff repair? A systematic review and meta-analysis study. European Journal of Orthopaedic Surgery and Traumatology. 2018;**28**(4):593-605. DOI: 10.1007/s00590-018-2145-7

[85] Chen M, Xu W, Dong Q, Huang Q, Xie Z, Mao Y. Outcomes of single-row versus double-row arthroscopic rotator cuff repair: A systematic review and meta-analysis of current evidence. Orthopedics. 2013;**29**(8):1437-1449. DOI: 10.1016/j.arthro.2013.03.076

[86] Yang J, Robbins M, Reilly J, Maerz T, Anderson K. The clinical effect of a rotator cuff retear: A meta-analysis of arthroscopic single-row and double-row repairs. The American Journal of Sports Medicine. 2017;**45**(3):733-741

[87] Mazzocca AD, Millett PJ, Guanche CA, Santangelo SA, Arciero RA. Arthroscopic single-row versus double-row suture anchor rotator cuff repair. The American Journal of Sports Medicine. 2005;**33**(12):1861-1868

[88] Kim DH, ElAttrache NS, Tibone JE, et al. Biomechanical comparison of a single-row versus double-row suture anchor technique for rotator cuff repair. The American Journal of Sports Medicine. 2006;**34**(3):407-414

[89] Baums MH, Spahn G, Buchhorn GH, Schultz W, Hofmann L, Klinger H-M. Biomechanical and magnetic resonance imaging evaluation of a single- and double-row rotator cuff repair in an in vivo sheep model. Arthroscopy. 2012;**28**(6):769-777

[90] Burkhart SS, Adams CR, Burkhart SS, Schoolfield JD. A biomechanical comparison of 2 techniques of footprint reconstruction for rotator cuff repair: The SwiveLock-FiberChain construct versus standard double-row repair. Arthroscopy. 2009;**25**(3):274-281

[91] Ma CB, Comerford L, Wilson J, Puttlitz CM. Biomechanical evaluation of arthroscopic rotator cuff repairs: Double-row compared with single-row fixation. The Journal of Bone and Joint Surgery. American Volume. 2006;**88**(2):403

[92] Christoforetti JJ, Krupp RJ, Singleton SB, Kissenberth MJ, Cook C, Hawkins RJ. Arthroscopic suture bridge transosseus equivalent fixation of rotator cuff tendon preserves intratendinous blood flow at the time of initial fixation. Journal of Shoulder and Elbow Surgery. 2012;**21**(4):523-530

[93] Cho NS, Lee BG, Rhee YG. Arthroscopic rotator cuff repair using a suture bridge technique: Is the repair integrity actually maintained. The American Journal of Sports Medicine. 2011;**39**(10):2108-2116

[94] Hayashida K, Tanaka M, Koizumi K, Kakiuchi M. Characteristic retear patterns assessed by magnetic resonance imaging after arthroscopic double-row rotator cuff repair. Arthroscopy. 2012;**28**(4):458-464

[95] Cho NS, Yi JW, Lee BG, Rhee YG. Retear patterns after arthroscopic rotator cuff repair: Single-row versus suture bridge technique. The American Journal of Sports Medicine. 2010;**38**(4):664-671

[96] Lee KW, Seo DW, Bae KW, Choy WS. Clinical and radiological evaluation after arthroscopic rotator cuff repair using suture bridge technique. Clinics in Orthopedic Surgery. 2013;**5**(4):306

[97] Kim KC, Shin HD, Cha SM, Park JY. Comparisons of retear patterns for 3 arthroscopic rotator cuff repair methods. The American Journal of Sports Medicine. 2014;**42**(3):558-565

Chapter 4

Fast Recovery in Esthetic Body Contouring Surgery

Héctor Durán, Lazaro Cardenas Camarena, Jorge Bayter, Juan Carlos Zambrano, Marcelo Uriarte and Alejandro López Echaury

Abstract

Body contouring surgery is worldwide accepted as one of the most successful esthetic surgeries. Lipectomy, liposuction, and buttock fat infiltration are among the most frequent procedures realized, but also, they are not free of complications as any other surgery. A strategy to overcome these complications is to provide the patient with a good perioperative care, to improve every aspect of recovery. The areas to be improved are nutrition, immunology, pain and inflammation, hemodynamics, early mobilization, patient education and communication, and leadership to evaluate if it is correctly been done. The implementation of these fast recovery strategies is the best approach for our patients, with cost-efficiency optimization, a better experience, and a high overall satisfaction during the whole process. It constitutes a paradigm shift from the traditional steps around the well-being of the patient. If all the areas are covered and improved, the patient should have a fast recovery and a good experience of the surgery.

Keywords: body contouring surgery, fast recovery, enhanced recovery in esthetic surgery, esthetic body contouring

1. Introduction

A surgery is an intervention that generates damage in an area of the human body in order to obtain a greater good. In cosmetic surgery, the objective of this controlled damage is to obtain greater beauty. But for this to happen, the damage will have to be controlled so that the body can recover. These procedures are usually performed on patients who must have optimal medical conditions. Therefore, recovery should be quick and smooth and is very desirable in all surgeries, especially in body contouring surgery. The goals of this work are to:

- share strategies to provide high quality indications, innovating in perioperative care [1];
- provide guidelines for a patient's rapid recovery;
- reduce the risk and frequency of complications from body contouring surgery [2]; and
- reduce hospitalization costs through a fast recovery.

2. Main text

According to ISAPS latest global report, body contouring surgeries (BCS) are among the top four procedures worldwide [3], with a tendency to increase every year; different techniques and technologies have been implemented to optimize the surgical act and improve the patient's esthetic outcome [4]. We recently searched for literature and realized that we could not find anything specific about optimizing the perioperative management in BCS, although we found some for breast augmentation and microvascular reconstruction [5, 6]. Therefore, we must first understand the problems and complications derived from BCS (mainly lipectomy and liposuction with buttock fat infiltration). By knowing the complications, we can develop strategies to prevent, mitigate, or avoid these complications. Fortunately, there are well-defined strategies for other surgery protocols, which can be used since they present similar complications [7].

The principles we used to select these strategies were that they could be grouped by systems (to facilitate their management), have a defined objective and scientific support, without interacting with the other recommendations, are cost-effective, and are easy to understand for patients. Based on the above principles, we consider that some points are highly relevant to achieve this rapid recovery, and we identified the following seven areas:

- Nutrition
    - An excellent preoperative diet and a quick restart
- Immunology
    - An adequate immunological function to decrease infections
- Pain and inflammation
    - Avoiding pain with strategies that promote comfort and mobility
- Hemodynamics
    - Hydration and response to bleeding, preventing thrombosis
- Early mobilization
    - To avoid complications and rapid reintegration
- Education and communication
    - Adequate patient education for active participation
- Leadership
    - Effective decision making and re-evaluation for improvement

3. Nutrition

Body contouring surgeries sometimes require more than 3 hours of surgical time, management of large surgical areas, and a large exchange of fluids (as in the case of liposculpture). Therefore, it is important to consider the management of perioperative nutrition as a fundamental pillar for a good recovery, as well as the multimodal management [2, 5–8]. Some of the possible benefits of adequate perioperative nutrition management such as decreased perioperative anxiety and thirst, controlled nausea and vomiting, decreased morbidity and mortality, and shortened hospital stay have been reported in different protocols [2, 5, 7, 9].

3.1 Preoperative management

In order to properly apply the recommendations, a patient undergoing body contouring surgery must be selected according to specific parameters [4] and preferably without comorbidities. Increased metabolic stress and insulin resistance are closely associated with fasting long periods [10], which may result in nausea, vomiting, and increased morbidity and mortality, including prolonged hospital stay and longer recovery period [1]; there are several perioperative guidelines and protocols published in order to avoid them [5, 6, 8]. In the case of body contouring surgeries, they are particularly useful and can be divided into:

- perioperative nutrition;
- fast to solid food; and
- fluid and carbohydrate loading.

3.2 Perioperative nutrition

The patient who undergoes elective body contouring surgeries must comply with the specific indications to improve his postoperative period, optimize recovery times, provide optimal conditions for healing, and prevent possible complications. Obese patients can also be malnourished; we suggest a complete nutritional evaluation, and the patient follows the appropriate and specific indications before surgery [9]. It is important to work on the patient's good eating habits and physical activity, since obesity is undoubtedly a factor that increases perioperative morbidity and mortality, wound dehiscence and infections, venous thromboembolism, and other complications. We would even recommend the surgeon to postpone surgery if the patient's weight is not adequate, seeking to perform elective surgeries on body mass indexes below 30 kg/m^2 ideally [11, 12]. It is important to integrate a group of professionals that includes a nutritionist and a psychologist, working together to improve our patient's behaviors and bad habits.

Alcoholic beverages should also be avoided. An intake of five or more alcoholic beverages in 1 day or five or more days in the last 30 days is considered high consumption and should be recommended to be suspended 1 month before surgery, since it is considered a risk factor frequently associated with wound infection [11].

Adequate preoperative intake should be monitored, and foods rich in protein and energy can be recommended 7 to 10 days before surgery [13, 14]. Supplements rich in arginine, fatty acids, and nucleotides have been shown to be effective in improving tissue oxygenation by promoting healing and overall recovery [13].

3.3 Preoperative fasting

Preoperative fasting is intended to prevent perioperative bronchoaspiration, which has a relatively low incidence but high mortality [15]. But fasting along with surgery can trigger increased insulin resistance and catabolic stress. Catabolic stress produces homeostasis alterations leading to an increase in the occurrence of nausea, vomiting, pain, and general postoperative discomfort that prolongs hospital stay [5, 13].

To avoid this, we recommend patients with BCS, a 6-hour fast for solid foods may be considered. Patients with underlying gastroduodenal pathology [5, 13, 14] and with evidence of delayed gastric emptying will need an 8-hour fast or an overnight fast.

Preoperative administration of carbohydrates (loading) is an option that should be considered 2 hours before the procedure and may be administered in clear liquids (maltodextrin, 12.5%, 285 mOsm/kg, 800 ml the evening before surgery and 400 ml 2–3 hours before induction of anesthesia) [5, 8, 9, 14]. In patients with delayed gastric emptying, carbohydrate loading should be avoided. These measures have been reported to decrease preoperative anxiety, in addition to suppressing thirst and postoperative discomfort [13, 14].

3.4 Postoperative nutritional management

Resuming an early oral intake after major surgery has shown many benefits, such as decreased nausea, faster return of bowel motility, and shorter hospital stay. It is generally recommended to start 4 hours after surgery, preferably with a low-residue diet. The addition of high-calorie and high-protein supplements will compensate for post-metabolic surgical stress [14].

Undoubtedly, nutrition is an important factor in improving critical postoperative aspects such as wound healing and infection prevention [5, 8, 13, 16]. Once the patient is at home, it is important to start a diet with supplementation of amino acids such as arginine and glutamine in addition to fatty acids, antioxidants, and nucleotides, since these are the most necessary nutrients for the body's metabolic response to surgical stress.

Several studies attribute benefits to arginine supplementation, which is associated with an improvement in vasodilation and oxygenation, in addition to normalizing T-lymphocyte function in tissues, enhancing the body's immune response, and accelerating biological recovery processes [13, 14].

Consuming protein-rich supplements has also been observed to reduce infection rate and hospital stay [13]. Similarly, supplementation with protein, iron, and vitamin B12 and supplementation with vitamin A, C, as well as zinc, calcium, and magnesium should be considered [17].

3.5 Reactivation of intestinal function

The consumption of coffee when started orally and gum (three times a day for 1 hour) has been widely studied to quickly reactivate the intestinal function, being these measures inexpensive and available in any recovery environment. Attempts have also been made to counteract the effect of opiates on intestinal motility by using alvimopan for its antagonistic effect on u-blockers in the gastrointestinal tract, as well as mosapride and its serotonin agonist action to enhance recovery from ileus [5, 13].

4. Immunology

4.1 Antimicrobial prophylaxis

It is important to note that surgical infections are rare in body contouring procedures [11, 18, 19], but adequate prophylaxis covering both aerobic and anaerobic bacteria is mandatory [20].

The appropriate time for antibiotic administration, according to current guidelines, is intravenous administration 60 minutes before the surgical procedure. The use of first-generation cephalosporins (Cefazolin 1 g) is preferred because of its wide coverage, low cost, and low allergenic potential [20–22].

The administration of oral antibiotics in the subsequent postoperative period lacks scientific support to demonstrate its efficacy in preventing infections, and its role in eliminating intestinal bacterial flora can be questioned [11, 20, 22].

4.2 Surgical area decontamination

It is recommended to clean the skin with alcohol and chlorhexidine solutions to eliminate the bacterial flora. Its use decreases the presence of surgical site infection by up to 40%. Studies have shown that they are more effective compared to povidone-iodine [11].

Preoperative bathing with chlorhexidine-based soaps remains questionable [20]; however, it can be considered useful as BCS works in large surgical areas, and this theoretically allows for more adequate preparation before the surgical procedure [11, 21].

5. Pain

5.1 Prevention and treatment of pain

One of the pillars of the comprehensive approach to surgical patient recovery is the management of analgesia. With this in mind, the first step is precisely to establish an appropriate analgesia management scheme even before the procedure. There is evidence that reducing pain during the intraoperative and postoperative processes will allow patients to have a faster nutritional, psychological, and motor recovery [23]. Among the results, a significant decrease in postoperative pain from day 0 to day 3 has been found. Another reason within rapid recovery protocols is to limit the use of opiates, thereby achieving the goal without increasing complications. On the other hand, opioids reduction is also part of the postoperative strategy to limit nausea and vomiting and avoid postural hypotension. These symptoms are a common cause of longer hospitalizations [11, 23, 24]. Among the recommendations for postoperative analgesia, treatment with ketorolac and then with paracetamol, nonsteroidal anti-inflammatory drugs, and gabapentin are recommended [25, 26].

Multimodal management is chosen to act on the different pain mechanisms and thus reduce them in the postoperative period [25]. As preoperative planning, celecoxib (200–400 mg), gabapentin (300–600 mg), and ondansetron (8 mg) are started as premedication one night before surgery and the surgery morning. Intraoperatively, dexamethasone (8 mg) and promethazine (25 mg) are added after induction, either intravenously or in suppository [26], in addition to fentanyl and propofol per kilogram of weight [23]. In breast surgery, the protocols also include regional anesthesia by paravertebral blocks [25] and in abdominoplasty the use of liposomal bupivacaine [27] (0.25–0.5%) below the rectus abdominis sheath [25] or transverse abdominal plane block. Ropivacaine as a pain control measure within the breast pocket in breast surgeries has also been reported efficiently by Durán-Vega [28]. In all cases, 1 g of paracetamol is applied intravenously at the end of surgery and just before extubation. In the recovery area, gabapentin can be used before discharge or during the hospital stay. For outpatient management, celecoxib and gabapentin are indicated for 5 to 7 days (**Table 1**) [26].

Moment	Drug
Night before surgery	Celecoxib
	Gabapentin
	Ondansetron
Morning of surgery	Celecoxib
	Gabapentin
	Ondansetron
Induction	Dexamethasone
	Promethazine (suppository)
Intraoperative	Acetaminophen
	Bupivacaine injection or ropivacaine pocket irrigation site (Duran's technique) [28]
Recovery	Gabapentin
Postoperative	Acetaminophen
	Celecoxib
	Gabapentin
	Methylprednisolone
	Tramadol (rescue)

Table 1.
Options for pain management.

6. Hemodynamics

The accelerated recovery protocol after surgery originated in the 1990s after findings from major research groups in elective surgery [29] demonstrated improved hydration, reduced incidence of bleeding, transfusions, and complications of thrombosis [1].

The strategies carried out in the perioperative period emphasize the application of management in the different stages of surgery, and one of the main objectives is to avoid the non-rational use of fluids to avoid water overload [30]. It has been shown that water overload is one of the main risk factors that increase morbidity and mortality. Inadequate use of intravenous fluids in quality and quantity favors tissue edema, increased body weight, and fluid leakage into the third space. This also translates into cardiorespiratory complications and, at abdominal level, into a delay in the recovery of adequate peristalsis, since it favors the presence of mesenteric edema and ascites.

Fluid restriction and the use of adequate intravenous fluids have resulted in less interstitial and visceral edema; however, the beneficial effects of such water restriction have not been fully demonstrated through various studies. Some meta-analyses even concluded that there is no decrease in complications or hospital stay [31]. Other randomized controlled studies report a decrease of up to 59% in complications in abdominal surgeries [32]. Optimizing water balance begins with the intake of clear liquids up to 2 hours before surgery [32]. Regarding solid food, it is recommended to be 6 hours before surgery.

But what is the volume that they consider ml/kg/hour within the (non-standardized) definition of water restriction? The range is from 4 to 9 ml/kg/hour compared to non-restriction of 18 ml/kg/hour. It is also important to consider the type and quality of the liquids used for a proper hydroelectrolyte balance ideally with balanced crystalloid solutions instead of saline solutions. Most of the studies are still inconclusive in this topic. Some multicenters report a 20% decrease in postoperative complications and others report a 40% decrease. However, a key element in the success of trans- and postsurgical care continue being continuous hemodynamic monitoring, including surveillance of variables as simple as urine volume per hour, being a very effective and minimally invasive tool. Hydration must always adjust the insensitive losses and the blood losses with crystalloids in each surgical procedure. It is recommended to keep IV fluids at a rate of 6 to 8 ml/kg/hour, the mean arterial pressure above 60 mmHg and the urinary output greater than 0.5 ml/kg/hour.

Patients treated with target-administered fluid therapy (TAFT) has shown in meta-analysis significantly lower morbidity ($p = 0.002$); therefore, the decrease in hospital stay, hospital costs, as well as lower mortality specifically due to major cardiovascular complications, in this case without being statistically significant ($p = 0.370$). It was demonstrated in all cases that managed with TAFT globally, less intraoperative fluids were administered compared to their controls [33]. We all recognize the need to replace water in surgery; however, the exact amount for a given procedure remains unknown, and the ideal volume should be identified in an attempt to avoid postoperative complications. Optimal management using conventional heart rate, blood pressure, and urine output parameters is difficult; so, TAFT was proposed; however, the beneficial effect is inconsistent. Nevertheless, TAFT is currently recommended in the context of protocols to improve postoperative recovery. The use of vasopressors is recommended to support fluid management and has no negative effect in the case of free flap surgery [12].

Regarding bleeding, studies by Zakhaleva and others, relate the use of less fluid, with less surgical morbidity [34]. Hemoglobin before surgery should ideally be greater than 13 g/dl [35] in an attempt to decrease morbidity and mortality from bleeding in our elective surgeries. In the case of anemia identified preoperatively, it should be corrected regardless of whether the cause is due to iron deficiency or some previously unidentified disorder [36].

Every patient will prove to be a different challenge in relation to bleeding. This can be related to factors like age, sex, medical history, comorbidities, type and duration of surgery, intraoperative and especially postoperative bleeding, drains use, etc. Also, anesthesia-related factors will have to be analyzed, such as hemodynamic monitoring technique, hemodynamic optimization, and fluid infusion solutions selected, among others [37].

The protocolization of the approach to fluid management will result in adequate perioperative water management, which will reduce costs, morbidity, and mortality, as well as the prompt recovery of our patients, avoiding high rates of postoperative morbidity and mortality dependent on water management by the anesthesiologist [38].

A fundamental element for the prevention of complications and an adequate perioperative evolution is venous thromboembolism prophylaxis. This becomes more relevant when the surgery includes abdominoplasty, a surgery that is usually known to have a higher risk of deep vein thrombosis and pulmonary embolism [18]. In these cases, it is essential to carry out a risk scale from the first contact in the office before elective surgery. There are several scales, and each team must determine which is the most appropriate to work with, although the best known is the scale of Caprini and Davidson [39]. The use of low-molecular-weight heparins is recommended in high-risk patients, unless the procedure is contraindicated and there is a high risk of postoperative bleeding. Among prophylactic measures, the use of graduated compression stockings, as well as intermittent mechanical pneumatic compression devices until the patient's discharge, is confirmed in different meta-analyses. Early ambulation is undoubtedly one of the main objectives of the rapid recovery process. Mobilization within the first 24 hours after the end of surgery is imperative.

7. Early mobilization

Early mobilization after any surgery is the key to rapid recovery from any surgery. This is desirable even in those surgeries where such mobilization would normally be thought to be contraindicated (for example, in the case of skin grafting) [40]; but in the case of body contouring surgery, mobilization is highly indicated. It is considered the most important general care measure in postoperative care to avoid complications [41]. Early mobilization also reduces hospital stay and hospitalization costs and improves the psychological well-being of patients; it promotes circulation, improves muscle tone, adds coordination and independence, improves bowel and urinary functions, and reduces the risk of pulmonary embolism and pneumonia. We owe this knowledge to Dr. Canavarro since World War II, who made the wounded walk from day 1, reporting a 50% reduction in complications in general [40].

Complications from not having early mobilization include muscle weakness, predisposition to lower extremity thrombosis and embolism, and impaired lung function [42]. For this reason, it is always desirable for the patient to move quickly. Also, mobilization is in full relation with the rest of the indications. For example, if anesthesia does not result in adequate recovery, the patient will not be able to mobilize properly. Or if the patient is in a lot of pain, mobilization will be extremely restricted. Similarly, nausea, cold, and other factors may prevent early mobilization.

One of the fears any doctor may have after surgery is that early mobilization will cause more bleeding. However, studies have shown that it is possible and indicated after surgeries even though when the risk of bleeding is thought to be higher. Southwell showed that there was neither any difference in graft integration nor was it necessarily associated with a higher risk of bruising, bleeding, infection, or slower integration [40]. Similarly, Yang after reconstructions [43] with maxillofacial free flap, considered mobilization as safe and that it could even have a better impact on patient comfort and sleep. Shakil [44] after orthopedic surgeries demonstrated that mobilization is not only desirable but also necessary, as it significantly reduces the rate of wound infection. Miyamoto [45] showed that early mobilization is possible after free anastomosis of the lower limbs. And Krauss [46] mentioned that in patients after hip arthroplasty surgery, it is possible to use tranexamic acid as an adjuvant to prevent bleeding and promote early mobilization.

8. Education and communication

A very important element is the adequate communication and information of patients through education and counseling of patients throughout the perioperative process. Human, physical, and digital resources can be used for this purpose. Knowing the complete perioperative procedure will help the patient to make the best decisions and to prepare physically and mentally in an adequate way for the surgery, as well as to know the process that will be presented during the recovery phase that starts from the postoperative recovery area.

Within this information, it is fundamental to inform the aspects that can interfere in the evolution and the result of the surgery, as well as those elements and factors that can increase the risk of some complications. The patient must change or suspend some behaviors like the habit of smoking, suggesting the complete abstinence from tobacco, both actively and passively, 4 weeks before the date of the surgery and at least 4 weeks after surgery [11].

Education and information about the perioperative process will allow the patient to collaborate with behaviors and attitudes that seek early recovery and the best outcome, since they will understand in detail the key elements that can prevent complications. The patient must know the importance of immediate ambulation (within the first 24 hours after surgery), the need and procedure for physical therapy, and postoperative rehabilitation.

Immediate postoperative follow-up with clear and precise indications and recommendations promotes early physical and emotional recovery. Adequate follow-up have been shown to promote better mobility, decrease pain scales, and promote the overall quality of life in the recovery process [47]. Appropriate follow-up includes supervised physical activation programs and other care and support initiatives to be implemented after discharge, which have been shown to accelerate recovery and mobility and improve patient self-confidence [48].

The central objective of educating a patient about the process he will face in surgery will be to have a proactive patient who understands what is happening. This patient will be able to differentiate between what is normal and what is not and will know the alarm data so that he can communicate with the surgeon on time in case of any eventuality. This will allow the surgeon to avoid or treat complications in a timely manner thanks to the cooperation of the patient, eliminating ignorance as an impediment to timely treatment.

9. Team leader and follow-up

For the correct application of these protocols, it is essential to establish a lead director of the indications, who within his functions will also ensure the socialization and compliance with the steps, and will monitor and establish the improvements or changes necessary for each group. Therefore, it is of great importance that the processes and successes are audited by a professional and multidisciplinary team [27].

As a major milestone, it is proposed that the patient can be discharged when the following conditions are met: oral fluid and solid tolerance, audible peristalsis, controllable pain with oral medications, assisted or independent mobilization, and absence of complications requiring hospitalization [27].

Rapid recovery protocols after surgery have shown that, even with variable surgeries and different populations, perioperative care determines outcome and success more than the surgical procedure itself [18]. The principles of these practices allow shorter stays and early mobility without increased morbidity [27]. Despite the numerous reports and solid literature on the benefits of rapid recovery protocols, differences in populations and access to resources and elements described above, patient comorbidities [27] involving behavioral changes among so many other variables should be identified by the team leader who should be sensitive to these differences and seek a solution for the different usual scenarios.

Lack of willingness to implement changes, non-standardization of processes and the execution without inspectors [49] are barriers that prevent the proper implementation of these strategies. For this reason, it is very important to be a leader who can work with barriers, such as general resistance to change, lack of time and team availability, and poor communication, collaboration, and coordination between departments [50].

10. Conclusion

The implementation of these fast recovery strategies is the best approach for our patients, with cost-efficiency optimization, a better experience, and a high overall satisfaction during the whole process [27]. It constitutes a paradigm shift from the traditional steps [24] around the well-being of the patient. It is possible to develop a management protocol that, although standardized, can be adapted to the different surgical groups performing BCS. In the area of nutrition, appropriate support should be sought to adequately nourish the patient so that the patient can have the least amount of fasting and a rapid tolerance to food. In the area of immunology, care must be taken to ensure that the patient has adequate immunological competence to keep inflammation under control and reduce infectious complications. Maintaining and taking care of an adequate hemodynamic function will help to avoid problems of postural hypotension, besides taking care of hemorrhage and adequate hydration, without it being minor or major. In the area of pain, try to make the patient feel as little discomfort as possible so that he or she can move and recover. Early mobilization will bring immediate benefits to the entire body. Proper patient education will help you understand the challenges you will face and communicate properly with the team to achieve a rapid response and avoid complications. And having a team leader who monitors the processes and implements the changes needed to make them truly effective will give the patient success for rapid recovery after BCS.

Acknowledgements

We would like to acknowledge Dra. Diana Cecilia Popoca for the translation of this document.

Conflict of interest

None of the authors declare any conflict of interest.

Author details

Héctor Durán[1,2,3,4,5,6]*, Lazaro Cardenas Camarena[1,2,3,4,6], Jorge Bayter[6,7,8,9,10,11], Juan Carlos Zambrano[5,12], Marcelo Uriarte[13,14] and Alejandro López Echaury[2,3,4]

1 ASAPS – American Society for Aesthetic Plastic Surgery, New York, USA

2 ASPS – American Society of Plastic Surgeons, Illinois, USA

3 AMCPER – Asociación Mexicana de Cirugía plástica estetica y reconstructive, Mexico

4 FILACP – Federación Ibero Latino Americana de Cirugía Plástica, Panama City, Panama

5 SAPS – South American Plastic Surgery, Bogota, Colombia

6 LATAM Safety Task Force is a Mexico-Colombia Union 14 FACS is Fellow of American College of Surgeons, USA

7 Universidad Industrial de Santander, Colombia

8 Reanimation Critical and Intensive Care, Universidad la Sabana in Bucaramanga, Colombia

9 Society of Ambulatory Anesthesia (SAMBA), Overland Park, Kansas

10 Colombian Society of Anesthesia and Reanimation (SCARE), Bogota, Colombia

11 Clínica "EL Pinar", Colombia

12 Pontificia Universidad Javeriana, Bogota, DC, Colombia

13 Uriarte Aesthetics, La Paz, Bolivia

14 FACS

*Address all correspondence to: hcdv@hotmail.com

References

[1] Bartlet EL, Zavlin D, Friedman JD. Enhanced recovery after surgery; the plastic surgery paradigm shift. Aesthetic Surgery Journal. 2018;**38**(6):676-685

[2] Ljungqvist O, Scott M, Fearon KC. Enhanced recovery after surgery: A review. JAMA Surgery. 2017;**152**(3):292-298

[3] International Society of Aesthetic Plastic Surgeons. ISAPS Global Survey Report. 2018. Available from: https://www.isaps.org/wp-content/uploads/2019/12/ISAPS-Global-Survey-Results-2018-new.pdf

[4] Ahmad J, Eaves FF III, Rohrich RJ, Kenkel JM. The American Society for Aesthetic Plastic Surgery (ASAPS) survey: Current trends in liposuction. Aesthetic Surgery Journal. 2011;**31**(2):214-224

[5] Batforf NJ, Lemaine V, Lovely JK, et al. Enhanced recovery after surgery in microvascular breast reconstruction. Journal of Plastic, Reconstructive & Aesthetic Surgery. 2015;**68**(3):395-402

[6] Dumestre DO, Webb CE, Temple-Oberle C. Improved recovery experience achieved for women undergoing implant-based breast reconstruction using an enhanced recovery after surgery model. Plastic and Reconstructive Surgery. 2017;**139**(3):550-559

[7] Kehlet H. Multimodal approach to control postoperative pathophysiology and rehabilitation. British Journal of Anaesthesia. 1997;**78**(5):606-617

[8] Fayezizadeh M, Petro CC, Rosen MJ, Novitsky YW. Enhanced recovery after surgery pathway for abdominal wall reconstruction: Pilot study and preliminary outcomes. Plastic and Reconstructive Surgery. 2014;**134** (4 Suppl 2):151S-159S

[9] Ljungqvist O, Jonathan E. Rhoads lecture 2011: Insulin resistance and enhanced recovery after surgery. JPEN Journal of Parenteral and Enteral Nutrition. 2012;**36**(4):389-398

[10] Bardram L, Funch-Jensen P, Jensen P, Crawford ME, Kehlet H. Recovery after laparoscopic colonic surgery with epidural analgesia, and early oral nutrition and mobilization. Lancet. 1995;**345**(8952):763-764

[11] Temple-Oberle C, Shea-Budgell MA, Tan M, Semple JL, Schrag C, Barreto M, et al. Consensus review of optimal perioperative care in breast reconstruction: Enhanced Recovery after Surgery (ERAS) Society recommendations. Plastic and Reconstructive Surgery. 2017;**139**(5):1056e-1071e. DOI: 10.1097/PRS.0000000000003242

[12] Lee KT, Mun GH. Effects of obesity on postoperative complications after breast reconstruction using free muscle-sparing transverse rectus abdominis myocutaneous, deep inferior epigastric perforator, and superficial inferior epigastric artery flap: A systematic review and meta-analysis. Annals of Plastic Surgery. 2016;**76**:576-584

[13] Van Der Hulst RR, van Kreel BK, von Meyenfeldt MF, et al. Glutamine and the preservation of gut integrity. Lancet. 1993;**342**(8857):1363-1365

[14] Nygren J, Thorell A, Jacobsson H, et al. Preoperative gastric emptying: Effects of anxiety and oral carbohydrate administration. Annals of Surgery. 1995;**222**(6):728-734

[15] Balteskard L, Unneberg K, Mjaaland M, Jenssen TG, Revhaug A. Growth hormone and insulin like growth factor 1 promote intestinal uptake and hepatic release of

glutamine in sepsis. Annals of Surgery. 1998;**228**(1):131-139

[16] Lassen K, Hannemann P, Ljungqvist O, et al. Patterns in current perioperative practice: Survey of colorectal surgeons in five northern European countries. BMJ. 2005;**330**(7505):1420-1421

[17] Thorell A, MacCormick AD, Awad S, et al. Guidelines for perioperative care in bariatric surgery: Enhanced Recovery After Surgery (ERAS) Society recommendations. World Journal of Surgery. 2016;**40**(9):2065-2083. DOI: 10.1007/s00268-016-3492-3

[18] Somogyi RB, Ahmad J, Shih JG, Lista F. Venous thromboembolism in abdominoplasty: A comprehensive approach to lower procedural risk. Aesthetic Surgery Journal. 2012;**32**(3):322-329. DOI: 10.1177/1090820X12438896

[19] Chia C, Neinstein R, Theodorou S. Evidence-based medicine: Liposuction. Plastic and Reconstructive Surgery. 2017;**139**(1):267e-274e

[20] Gustafsson UO, Scott MJ, Hubner M, et al. Guidelines for perioperative care in elective colorectal surgery: Enhanced Recovery After Surgery (ERAS®) Society recommendations: 2018. World Journal of Surgery. 2019;**43**(3):659-695

[21] Nelson G, Bakkum-Gamez J, Kalogera E, Altman A, Meyer LA, Scott M, et al. Guidelines for perioperative care in gynecologic/oncology: Enhanced Recovery after Surgery (ERAS) Society recommendations—2019 update. International Journal of Gynecological Cancer. 2019;**29**(4):651-668

[22] Melloul E, Lassen K, Roulin D, Grass F, Perinel J, Adham M, et al. Guidelines for perioperative care for pancreatoduodenectomy: Enhanced Recovery After Surgery (ERAS) recommendations. 2019. World Journal of Surgery. 2020. ISO 690

[23] Dumestre DO, Redwood J, Webb CE, Temple-Oberle C. Enhanced recovery after surgery (ERAS) protocol enables safe same-day discharge after alloplastic breast reconstruction. Plastic Surgery. 2017;**25**(4):249-254. DOI: 10.1177/2292550317728036

[24] Offodile AC, Gu C, Boukovalas S, et al. Enhanced recovery after surgery (ERAS) pathways in breast reconstruction: Systematic review and meta-analysis of the literature. Breast Cancer Research and Treatment. 2019;**173**(1):65-77. DOI: 10.1007/s10549-018-4991-8

[25] Parikh RP, Myckatyn TM. Paravertebral blocks and enhanced recovery after surgery protocols in breast reconstructive surgery: Patient selection and perspectives. Journal of Pain Research. 2018;**11**:1567-1581. DOI: 10.2147/JPR.S148544

[26] Bartlett EL, Zavlin D, Friedman JD, Abdollahi A, Rappaport NH. Enhanced recovery after surgery: The plastic surgery paradigm shift. Aesthetic Surgery Journal. 2018;**38**(6):676-685. DOI: 10.1093/asj/sjx217

[27] Jogerst K, Thomas O, Kosiorek HE, et al. Same-day discharge after mastectomy: Breast cancer surgery in the era of ERAS®. Annals of Surgical Oncology. 2020. DOI: 10.1245/s10434-020-08386-w

[28] Durán-Vega HC, Ramírez-Montañana A, Galindo OG, Gutierrez AM, González AZ, Galindo EG, et al. Ropivacaine in breast augmentation surgery. Plastic and Reconstructive Surgery. Global Open. 2018;**6**(5):1-4

[29] de Jesús Sánchez-Zúñiga M. Medicina Crítica. 2016;**39**(Suppl 1):10-14

[30] Carrillo-Esper R, de los Monteros-Estrada E, Pérez-Calatayud A. Una nueva propuesta de la medicina perioperatoria. El protocolo ERAS. Revista Mexicana de Anestesiología. 2013;**36**(S1):296-301

[31] Abraham-Nordling M, Hjern F, Pollack J, Prytz M, Borg T, Kressner U. Randomized clinical trial of fluid restriction in colorectal surgery. The British Journal of Surgery. 2012;**99**:186-191

[32] Brandstrup B, Tønnesen H, Beier-Holgersen R, et al. Effects of intravenous fluid restriction on postoperative complications: Comparison of two perioperative fluid regimens. A randomized assessor-blinded multicenter trial. Annals of Surgery. 2003;**238**:641-648

[33] Hamilton MA, Cecconi M, Rhodes A. A systematic review and meta-analysis on the use of preemptive hemodynamic intervention to improve postoperative outcomes in moderate and high-risk surgical patients. Anesthesia and Analgesia. 2011;**112**:1392-1402

[34] Zakhaleva J, Tam J, Denoya PI, Bishawi M, Bergamaschi R. The impact of intravenous fluid administration on complication rates in bowel surgery within an enhanced recovery protocol: A randomized controlled trial. Colorectal Disease. 2013;**15**:892-899

[35] Ripollés-Melchor J. Association between use of enhanced recovery after surgery protocol and postoperative complications in colorectal surgery: The postoperative outcomes within enhanced recovery after surgery protocol (POWER) study. JAMA Surgery. 2019;**154**(8):725-736

[36] Batchelor TJP, Rasburn NJ, Abdelnour-Berchtold E, Brunelli A, Cerfolio RJ, Gonzalez M, et al. Guidelines for enhanced recovery after lung surgery: Recommendations of the Enhanced Recovery After Surgery (ERAS®) Society and the European Society of Thoracic Surgeons (ESTS). European Journal of Cardio-Thoracic Surgery. 2019;**55**(1):91-115

[37] ERAS Compliance Group. The impact of enhanced recovery protocol compliance on elective colorectal cancer resection: Results from an international registry. Annals of Surgery. 2015;**261**:1153-1159

[38] Lagarda-Cuevas J. Terapia de líquidos dirigida por metas en cirugía mayor no cardíaca: metaanálisis y revisión de la literatura. 2018;**41**(2):105-116

[39] Cuenca-Pardo J, Ramos-Gallardo G, Morales Olivera M, Bucio-Duarte J, Caravantes-Cortés I. Stratification of the risk of thrombosis and prophylaxis: What is the best score to stratify the risk of thrombosis in patients of plastic surgery? What is the best prophylaxis? Evidence based medicine. Cirugía Plástica. 2020;**29**(1):32-47

[40] Southwell-Keely J, Vandervord J. Mobilisation versus bed rest after skin grafting pretibial lacerations: A meta-analysis. Plastic Surgery International. 2012;**2012**:1-6. DOI: 10.1155/2012/207452

[41] Morris BA, Benetti M, Marro H, Rosenthal CK. Clinical practice guidelines for early mobilization hours after surgery. Orthopaedic Nursing. 2010;**29**(5):290-316. DOI: 10.1097/NOR.0b013e3181ef7a5d

[42] Kitching AJ, O'Neill SS. Fast-track surgery and anaesthesia. Continuing Education in Anaesthesia Critical Care & Pain. 2009;**9**(2):39-43. DOI: 10.1093/bjaceaccp/mkp006

[43] Yang Y, Wu HY, Wei L, Li PJ, Cai ZG, Shan XF. Improvement of the patient early mobilization protocol

after oral and maxillofacial free flap reconstruction surgery. Journal of Cranio-Maxillofacial Surgery. 2020;**48**(1):43-48. DOI: 10.1016/j.jcms.2019.11.016

[44] Shakil S, Rehman U, Danish K. The role of early mobilization in the prevention of post operative wound infection after lower extremity orthopedic surgeries. Journal of the Islamic International Medical College. 2012;**7**(January):63-66

[45] Miyamoto S, Kayano S, Fujiki M, Chuman H, Kawai A, Sakuraba M. Early mobilization after free-flap transfer to the lower extremities: Preferential use of flow-through anastomosis. Plastic and Reconstructive Surgery Global Open. 2014;**2**(3):1-7. DOI: 10.1097/GOX.0000000000000080

[46] Krauss ES, Cronin MA, Suratwala SJ, Enker P, Rosen L, Segal A. Use of intravenous tranexamic acid improves early ambulation after total knee arthroplasty and anterior and posterior total hip arthroplasty. American Journal of Orthopedics (Belle Mead, N.J.). 2017;**46**(5):E314-E319

[47] Testa A, Iannace C, Di Libero L. Strengths of early physical rehabilitation programs in surgical breast cancer patients: Results of a randomized controlled study. European Journal of Physical and Rehabilitation Medicine. 2014;**50**:275-284

[48] Cho HS, Davis GC, Paek JE, et al. A randomised trial of nursing interventions supporting recovery of the postmastectomy patient. Journal of Clinical Nursing. 2013;**22**:919-929

[49] Ament SM, Gillissen F, Moser A, et al. Identification of promising strategies to sustain improvements in hospital practice: A qualitative case study. BMC Health Services Research. 2014;**14**(1):641

[50] Pearsall EA, Meghji Z, Pitzul KB, et al. A qualitative study to understand the barriers and enablers in implementing an enhanced recovery after surgery programs. Annals of Surgery. 2015;**261**(1):92-96

Chapter 5

Surgical Recovery of Intestinal Obstructions: Pre- and Postoperative Care and How Could it Be Prevented?

Burhan Hakan Kanat, Erhan Eröz, Atakan Saçli, Nizamettin Kutluer, Mehmet Gençtürk and Selim Sözen

Abstract

Although initial data on intestinal obstructions are based on Hippocrates, there is still no consensus on approaches today. However, parallel to the development of medical technology and the increasing experience of us surgeons, morbidity and mortality rates due to intestinal obstruction have decreased. Obstruction can occur at any point in the gastrointestinal tract. The main thing is to make a correct diagnosis and to treat the patient in the most correct way. Intestinal obstructions usually present with colic abdominal pain, nausea, vomiting, and constipation. Intestinal obstructions may be present due to various reasons. Surgeons have an important role in preventive mechanical obstructions due to adhesions. Patients must be hospitalized. If there is no emergency surgical indication, conservative methods can be applied. Patients should be mobilized early, and fluid-electrolyte balance should be adjusted and followed closely.

Keywords: intestinal obstructions, conservative methods, treatment

1. Introduction

Intestinal obstruction is a clinical manifestation that occurs since the passage of the intestinal contents, which should be into the distal levels, is prevented in any part of the passage. It is a condition frequently encountered in the emergency department, which gives positive results with early diagnosis and accurate treatment methods but may have negative consequences if it is not managed well. The patients usually present with the complaints of nausea and vomiting, colic abdominal pain, and inability to defecate. Intestinal obstruction accounts for 5–15% of the patients presenting to the emergency department with acute abdomen [1–3].

In parallel with the development of medical technology and the increasing experience of us, the surgeons, morbidity and mortality rates due to intestinal obstruction have decreased, but difficulties in diagnosis and treatment remain. Now, the cases may present with more complex conditions, and treatment may become more complicated. Nowadays, when minimally invasive and conservative methods are more popular, there is no doubt that nonoperative approach should be the preferred approach for intestinal obstruction. However, unfortunately, surgery should not be delayed, and appropriate intervention should be performed in the presence of a condition that requires absolute surgery in its etiology.

Obstruction can occur at any point in the gastrointestinal tract. Correct diagnosis and appropriate treatment of the patient is essential. Another important point, especially in surgical treatment, is to prevent brid formation which may cause re-obstruction. In addition, absolute oncological principles should be followed in obstructions caused by tumors, etc.

Intestinal obstructions can be due to very simple benign causes that need to be considered or malignant causes where no intervention apart from palliative surgical interventions can be performed [1–6]. Here, we will examine this entity with a wide clinical, treatment, and follow-up margin.

2. Etiology

Mechanical intestinal obstructions may be present due to various reasons. Etiology should be learned well to be able to determine the appropriate treatment option. The causes of intestinal obstruction can be broadly classified into three categories [3].

1. Intraluminal

2. Intramural

3. Extrinsic factors

Intraluminal causes can be defined as factors causing obstruction by not allowing intestinal passage. These can be exemplified as gallstones, foreign bodies such as bezoar, and solidified ileal content.

Tumors of the small intestine, inflammatory small bowel diseases such as Crohn's disease, intramural hematoma, invagination, and stricture due to radiotherapy can be considered as intramural causes.

This part, which is classified as extrinsic factors, appears more than the sum of the other two parts. We know that adhesions secondary to previous abdominal surgery account for approximately 75% of small intestinal obstructions. In addition, we encounter with a considerable amount of hernias, congenital anomalies, and carcinomatosis due to intra-abdominal tumors [7, 8].

According to the mechanism of formation, there are also paralytic ileus, spastic ileus, and chronic intestinal pseudo-obstruction as well as mechanical intestinal obstruction. While paralytic ileus can be observed as a result of insufficient nerve conduction due to excessive analgesic use or electrolyte imbalance, spastic ileus occurs in cases of increased nerve conduction, such as metal poisoning [2, 7–9].

3. Clinic

Small intestinal obstructions usually present with colic abdominal pain, nausea, vomiting, and constipation. If obstruction is at proximal levels, vomiting is more prominent, while if it is at distal levels, abdominal distension is more prominent. Although intestinal sounds, by listening, may increase in the early period, they decrease in later periods. Strangulation or ischemia should be considered if there is severe abdominal pain that is not correlated with mild distention, and the diagnosis and treatment should be made without any delay [9].

4. Diagnosis

Although it is known by the world of medicine that a good anamnesis is necessary for the diagnosis, it has been shown to be more important in the diagnosis of ileus. The presence of previous abdominal surgery and intra-abdominal disease (Crohn's disease, tumor, etc.) should be questioned in the anamnesis, and the inguinal region should be checked for hernias during the examination.

Plain abdominal radiography in the standing position should be first obtained for the radiological imaging of the patient. Plain radiography is an examination that has been used for about half a century. The radiograph should be checked for enlarged small intestinal loop and air-fluid level. If present, it should be noted whether this is from the small intestine or the large intestine (**Figures 1** and **2**). It should not be forgotten that obstructions proximal to the small intestine may be overlooked as they may not be able to produce air-fluid level on the radiograph. Nevertheless, it is still used as the cheapest, most practical, and easiest diagnostic method in appropriate patients [3, 10, 11].

Abdominal ultrasonography is an option that may be beneficial in cases where direct radiography is contraindicated such as pregnancy, although it is not in the first place in practice [3, 12].

Computed tomography has a sensitivity and specificity of approximately 80–90% in detecting small intestinal obstructions. Tomography may show the point causing small intestinal obstruction (transition zone), loss of diameter in large loops proximal to the transition zone and loops distal to the transition zone, and decompression in the colon due to lack of ileal content. Closed loop is visible, if present. Hematoma in the small intestinal wall, tumor, and invagination can also be observed if obstruction is due to an intramural cause. Gallstones, bezoars, and foreign bodies, which are among the intraluminal causes, can also be easily observed by computed tomography [10–12].

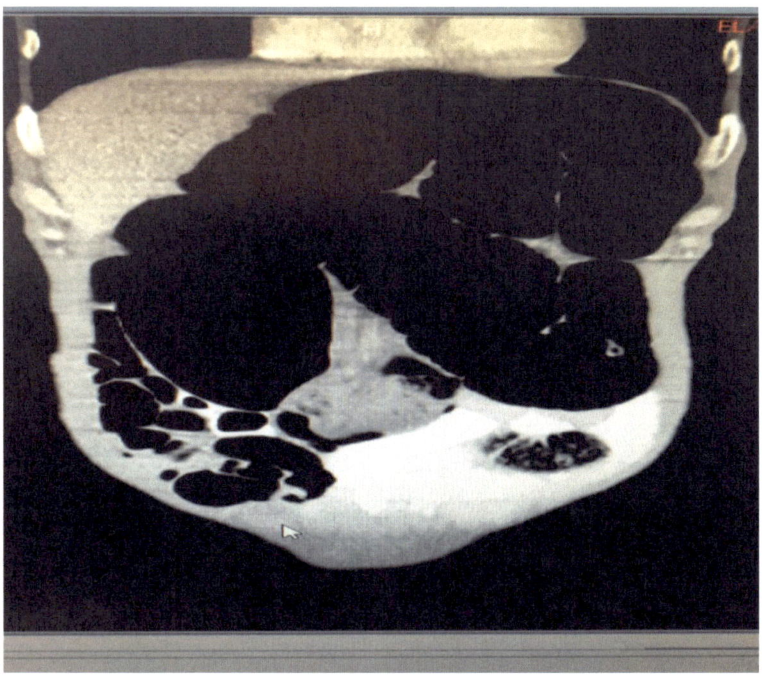

Figure 1.
Volvulus view on plain radiography (from the archive of Burhan Hakan Kanat).

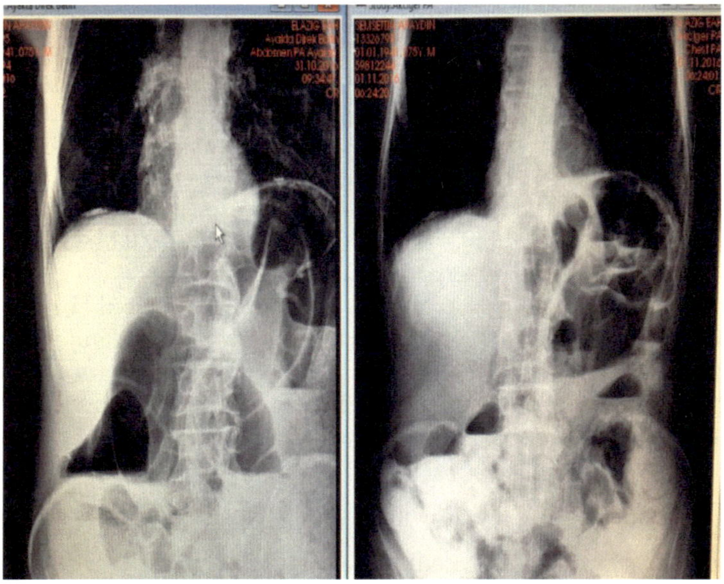

Figure 2.
Enlarged small intestinal loop and air-fluid levels in the radiograph (from the archive of Burhan Hakan Kanat).

In laboratory tests, it should be kept in mind that the patient may be in a hemoconcentrated state following the intravascular volume decrease due to fluid loss to the third space. Dehydration may occur due to loss of intravascular volume. Hypokalemic-hypochloremic metabolic alkalosis may occur depending on the severity of vomiting. Leukocytosis may be added to the condition due to bacterial translocation, and lactate may increase as a finding of ischemia in the presence of closed loop [2, 13, 14].

5. Treatment

Although some statements like "the sun should not rise" or "the sun should not set on the patient with the diagnosis of intestinal obstruction" have been made before, nonoperative approach is now applied to the patients with obstruction as in all areas of surgery. However, it should be kept in mind that complete obstruction and closed loop obstruction must be excluded for this approach [15].

Laboratory tests should be performed to see if there is an electrolyte imbalance. The dehydrated patient should be started on fluid therapy rapidly, and urinary catheter should be inserted to monitor urine output in the presence of additional diseases such as cardiac disorders. If necessary, central venous catheter insertion and CVP monitoring are among the treatment options for continuation of fluid therapy. When leukocytosis and CRP elevation are observed, prophylactic antibiotherapy should be started to prevent peritonitis secondary to bacterial translocation.

When air-fluid level is observed on standing plain abdominal radiograph, a nasogastric catheter should be inserted, and oral intake should be restricted. As a result of this decompression, aspiration, nausea, and vomiting can be prevented [16].

Computed tomography performed using water-soluble radiopaque materials such as gastrografin can show the location, characteristics of the obstruction, and whether complete obstruction occurred or not. Although it has not yet been proven in the literature, there are some authors who argue that gastrografin accelerating the passage inside the loop helps maintain local fluid-electrolyte balance.

After exclusion of closed loop and intestinal ischemia, the patient can be followed up with nonoperative approach. In this context, the presence of peritonitis and distention should be evaluated during regular abdominal examinations. Intermittent plain radiographs should be performed to see if the air-fluid levels seen in the first radiograph have decreased or replaced. Leukocyte and lactate values, gas-stool discharge, and nasogastric catheter flow rates should be closely monitored. Continuous mobilization of the patient during this follow-up reduces the length of hospital stay.

It was reported that no improvement was seen in approximately 5–15% of the patients within the first 48 h by nonoperative approach. Therefore, laparotomy option should be kept in mind for the patients who do not have significant improvement in their clinical findings after 48 h (**Figures 3** and **4**). It is known that the surgical decision taken after this 2-day waiting period does not increase mortality [17].

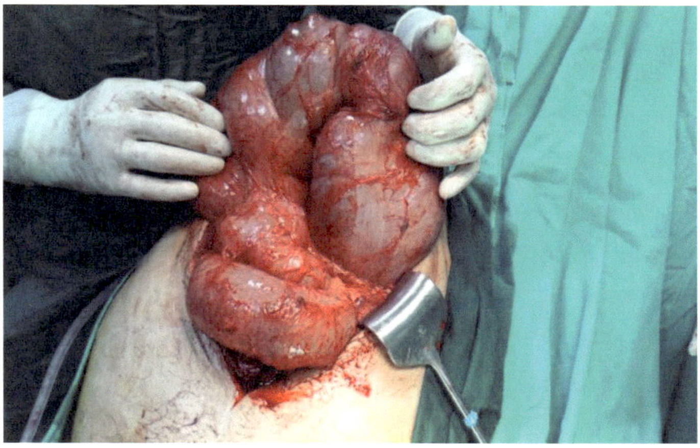

Figure 3.
Surgery image of a patient with volvulus (from the archive of Burhan Hakan Kanat).

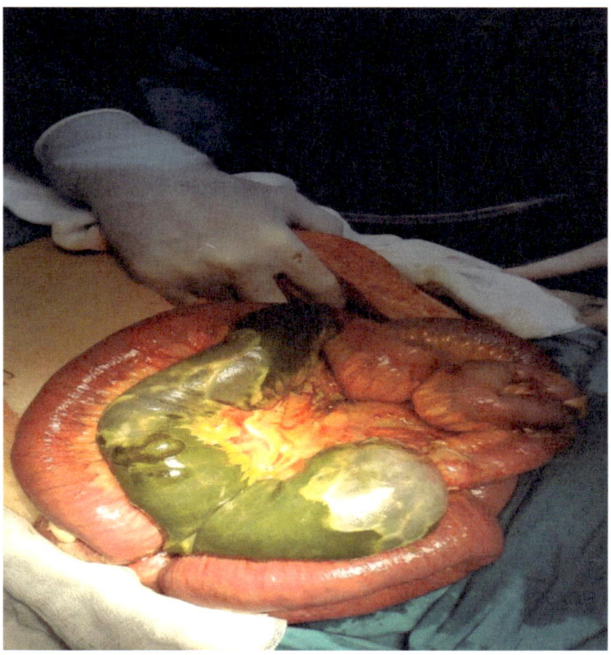

Figure 4.
Bowel loop gone to necrosis due to internal herniation (from the archive of Burhan Hakan Kanat).

With the decrease of nasogastric catheter flow rate and the onset of gas-stool discharge, NG catheter can be withdrawn first, oral intake can be started over time, and food intake can be gradually increased.

Although open surgical technique is found in the first place in practice, there are also studies showing that laparoscopic surgery can be performed in selected cases. Important parameters such as early diagnosis, proximal obstruction, partial obstruction, and the number of previous abdominal surgeries are available [18]. The algorithm can be followed in follow-up and treatment (Algorithm).

A. Algorithm

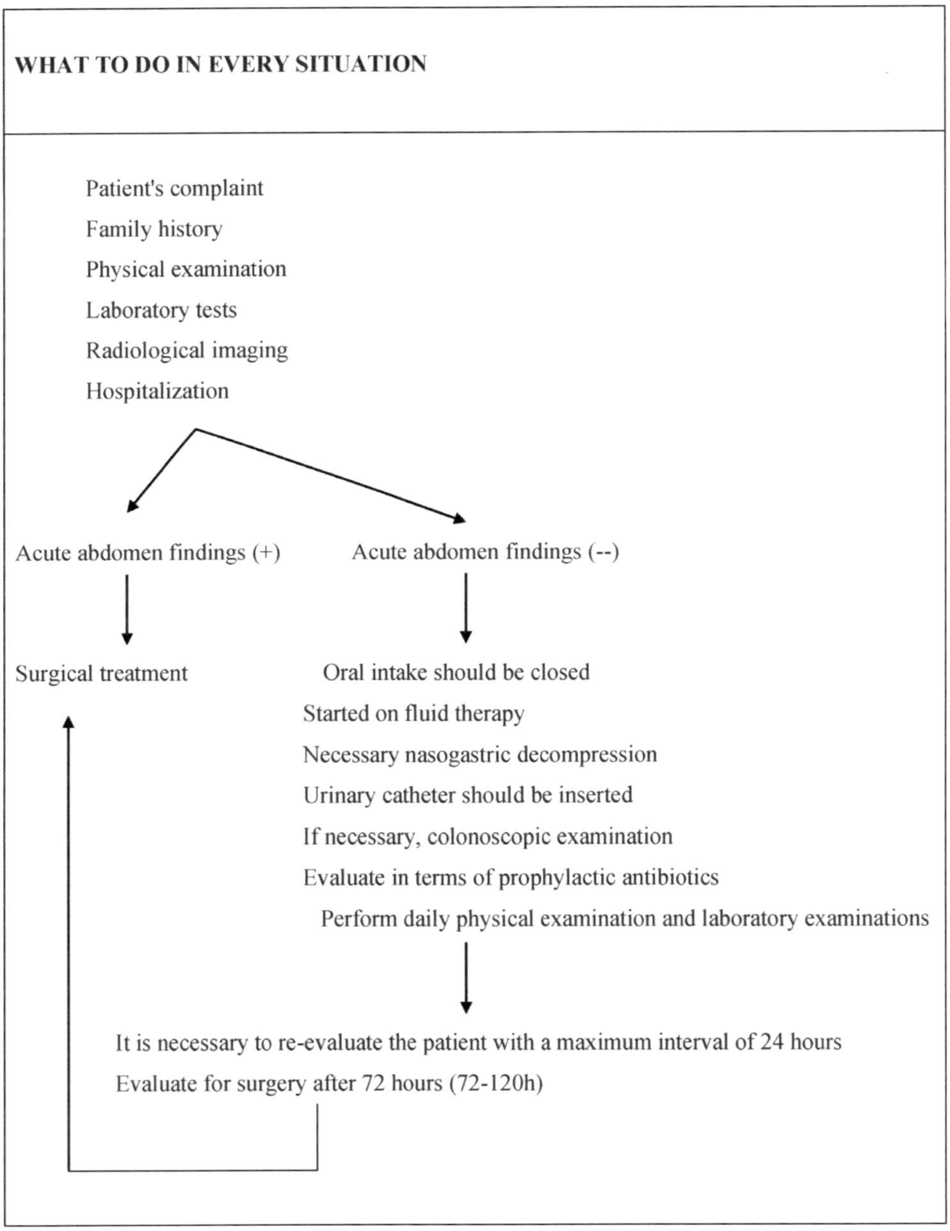

6. Postoperative care and prevention efforts

Surgeons have an important duty especially in preventable mechanical obstructions due to adhesions. It is needed to pay attention to surgical rules such as minimal touching the intestines during surgery, preferring laparoscopic surgical procedures if possible, and minimizing perioperative fluid resuscitation. Transition to early oral nutrition, minimal NSAID and opioid use, administration of epidural anesthesia if possible, avoiding excessive fluid resuscitation, and close monitoring of electrolytes should be taken into consideration in the postoperative period.

The main goal in the treatment of the patients with intestinal obstruction should be to prevent unnecessary surgeries. Peristalsis-increasing agents may be given to provide anal discharge of gas in the intestine if there is no contraindication (mechanical obstruction, etc.). It is needed to prevent the introduction and production of new gas into the intestine. It may be necessary to insert a nasogastric catheter to allow the introduction of atmospheric air and easy release of air refluxing in the stomach. Although the nasogastric catheter is not very comfortable for the patient, it is very useful in some patients.

Fluid-electrolyte balance can rapidly change in these patients. It is needed to be on the alert for this condition, and the patient should be closely followed up. Fluid-electrolyte imbalance is the most important pathology that prevents physiological gas absorption from the intestinal wall. If fluid-electrolyte imbalance is corrected quickly and accurately, intestinal mucosal cell functions will be improved, and therefore a large amount of CO_2 can be transferred through the lumen into the blood.

There are different approaches for some patients especially those with tumor-induced obstruction. Temporary ostomy and definitive surgery can be performed after bowel cleansing in order to keep patient comfort at a better level. Or appropriate surgery can be performed in a single session considering the general condition and additional diseases of the patient.

It is recommended to follow up some of the patients requiring surgery in the secondary or intensive care units in the postoperative period. There are important steps in early follow-up and treatment of the patients. Pulse rate, respiration rate, blood pressure, oxygen saturation, and body temperature should be closely monitored. There is no standard protocol for their monitoring frequency. Many clinics or intensive care units have standardized blood test monitoring. The laboratory values to be controlled are arranged depending on the factors such as size and duration of surgery, intraoperative interventions, renal functions, etc. Blood count, bleeding-coagulation panel, and renal and liver function tests are the most frequently studied parameters. The acid–base balance of the patient is also monitored, especially if the operation is prolonged. The patient's intake and discharge should be closely monitored, and fluid intake should be adjusted accordingly. Fluid-electrolyte balance is especially important [19].

In these patients, multimodal management of nausea and vomiting, use of nasogastric catheter, application of urinary catheter and withdrawal time, stimulation of gastrointestinal motility, appropriate analgesia, when to feed the patient, and especially early mobilization are important in the postoperative period [20, 21].

The application of nasogastric catheters was first performed by Levine and Paine to reduce nausea, vomiting, and distension occurring after abdominal surgery. It has continued to be used in the same way since those years. Although many recent studies do not recommend its routine use, a considerable number of surgeons apply it traditionally [22]. Nasogastric catheter poses risks in terms of both comfort and complications for patients.

Despite advances in surgical treatment methods and increased experience of surgeons, postoperative pain is the most common symptom experienced by patients and is a condition that adversely affects patient comfort. Postoperative pain has a negative effect on the quality of life of patient and prolongs the period of return to daily activities and hospital stay. Thus, it increases the cost. Postoperative pain management is an issue that needs to be meticulously addressed. It may cause anxiety both in patients and their relatives, especially in hospitalized patients. The aim of providing analgesia is to minimize or prevent the patient's discomfort, to protect against side effects, to reduce the length of hospital stay, and to prevent recurrence of pain complaints. Pharmacological and non-pharmacological methods are used in postoperative pain management [23, 24].

Malnutrition is one of the most important patient-related factors affecting morbidity and mortality in surgical patients. The most important step in nutrition is to identify the patient with malnutrition or the patient with the possibility of developing malnutrition. There are several screening methods for this. It is essential to provide adequate support when preparing the patient for surgery. Nutritional support can be provided by direct oral intake, enteral feeding tube, and parenteral route both preoperatively and postoperatively. Each alternative has its own advantages and disadvantages. Many hospitals have nutrition teams that follow up patients and provide adequate support. There are also some authors who argue that excessive feeding in the preoperative period triggers the risk of infection due to hyperglycemia [25].

Nutritional status of the patient should be closely monitored, and necessary support should be provided for early recovery. It is recommended to gradually start oral intake after sarcoma surgeries, if there is no intervention to the gastrointestinal organs. The preferred and recommended route is the enteral route as in any patient.

7. How can adhesions be prevented?

Every surgical intervention has a skin scar that appears from the outside. What about inside? Adhesion formation after surgery is inevitable but it is possible to minimize it. Minimally invasive surgery (robotic, laparoscopic, endoscopic), to which traditional open surgery is gradually giving way, can be considered as the first step to reduce adhesion formation. Minimally invasive surgery is very valuable in reducing brid formation by shortening the duration of surgery, eliminating intestinal contact, and reducing the amount of bleeding.

Bleeding during surgery and insufficient clearance of bleeding-related clots and inadequate intra-abdominal washing are predisposing factors for postoperative adhesions. On the other hand, the amount of contact with the intestines during abdominal surgery is correlated with brid formation.

Surgical planning should be made as soon as possible in infective pathologies (perforation, appendicitis, etc.). The elapsed waiting time will increase postoperative adhesion formation.

8. Conclusions

After surgery, intestinal function usually returns to normal within 5 days. If it persists for longer than this, it is considered a paralytic ileus. Recovering from an ileus depends on getting the proper treatment for the underlying cause. Ileus is a relatively common condition that is easy to treat. It is especially prevalent in those who have undergone recent abdominal or pelvic surgery. An awareness of the symptoms is key to improving the outlook and reducing the risk of complications. It is essential to seek prompt medical treatment as soon as symptoms appear.

The cornerstone of nonoperative management of small bowel obstruction caused by adhesions is starvation and stomach decompression using a nasogastric tube and fluid resuscitation. This approach seems uniform for younger and older patients. Nonoperative management should further include correction of electrolyte disturbances and nutritional support, especially in the frail older patient to avoid delirium, functional decline, and complications as a result of starvation and malnutrition. Nonoperative management is effective in approximately 70–90% of patients with adhesive small bowel obstruction in general. Though it has a significant failure rate, the nasogastric tube remains relevant in the conservative treatment of small bowel obstruction to initially relieve symptoms and avoid aspiration. An ongoing debate in the management of small bowel obstruction is the duration of nonoperative treatment that is deemed mandatory to resolve the bowel obstruction before the decision to operate. Most authors apply the 72-h safe-time rule for duration of initial nonoperative therapy irrespective of age [26–29].

9. Place of the endoscopy in acute conditions

The term acute mechanical intestinal obstruction describes the condition of preventing the progression of the contents in the intestinal lumen for mechanical reasons [30]. Complaints and clinical findings can be quite guiding in the diagnosis of obstruction and can be meaningless or misleading. The accuracy rate of direct abdominal X-ray in the diagnosis of obstruction is approximately 50–70% among the initial examinations of patients with acute abdominal pain. However, it is possible to say the level and degree of obstruction in diagnostic direct abdominal X-rays and even the presence of some complications (such as perforation) [31, 32]. Today, computed tomography is the gold standard imaging method. It not only makes a diagnosis but also provides important information on determining the etiological cause, determining the level and degree of obstruction, presence of strangulation, monitoring, and treatment [33, 34].

Emergency colonoscopy, which has recently become prominent in distal intestinal obstructions, offers important diagnostic and therapeutic opportunities. Although colonoscopic examination performed in emergency conditions is more likely to not be performed optimally or fails and requires more experience, it not only shows the cause, level, degree, and presence of ischemia in cases where it is successful but also enables endoscopic treatment [30–37]. There are many endoscopic methods used in the treatment of large bowel obstructions; the most preferred among these are procedures that reduce tumor size, tube administration, stenting, dilation, and detortion.

Endoscopic stenting is a frequently preferred method for both malignant and benign bowel obstructions. Stenting has two important advantages in malignant obstructions:

1. It is also known as bridging treatment, by eliminating the emergency, giving the patient the chance to perform elective surgery with much lower morbidity and mortality rates.

2. It provides palliation in patients with stage 4 disease or poor candidate for surgery, after the removal of the emergency after stenting, so that the patient does not have to live dependent on stoma in the remaining life [30].

Emergency colonoscopy should be in the first place for patients who are considered to have mechanical obstruction especially for the colon.

10. Pregnancy and intestinal obstruction

Although intestinal obstruction is rare in pregnancy, it is seen in the ratio of 1/10–16 thousand. Intestinal obstruction is most common in pregnancy at the beginning of the second trimester, at the end of pregnancy, and in the puerperium. The time of its appearance is parallel to the displacement of the intestines. Pregnancy can change or mask the signs and symptoms of the disease, so its diagnosis is more difficult [38, 39].

The most important cause of pregnancy intestinal obstructions is brids. Volvulus and intussusception are other common causes. It should be remembered that malignant and benign tumors can also be seen [40]. For diagnosis, abdominal ultrasonography should be the first choice since it does not contain radiation. If it is still preferred, computed tomography should be preferred instead of X-ray [39]. Colonoscopy may be preferred in patients who are considering volvulus. In treatment, surgery should be avoided as much as possible. However, there are the same treatment options as normal patients, if necessary [38].

Author details

Burhan Hakan Kanat[1], Erhan Eröz[2], Atakan Saçli[3], Nizamettin Kutluer[1], Mehmet Gençtürk[4] and Selim Sözen[5]*

1 Department of General Surgery, Health Sciences University, Elazig Fethi Sekin State Hospital, Elazig, Turkey

2 Department of General Surgery, Toyotasa Emergency Hospital, Sakarya, Turkey

3 Department of General Surgery, İskenderun State Hospital, Hatay, Turkey

4 Istanbul Obesity Surgery (IOC) Clinic, Kurtköy Ersoy Hospital, Istanbul, Turkey

5 Sözen Surgery Clinic, Istanbul, Turkey

*Address all correspondence to: selimsozen63@yahoo.com

References

[1] Macutkiewicz C, Carlson GL. Acute abdomen: Intestinal obstruction. Surgery (Oxford). 2008;**26**(3):102-107

[2] Jackson PG, Raiji MT. Evaluation and management of intestinal obstruction. American Family Physician. 2011;**83**: 159-165

[3] Tavakkoli A, Ashley SW, Zinner MJ. Small bowel obstruction: Section 28. In: Brunicardi FC, editor. Schwartz's Principles of Surgery. 10th ed. New York, USA: McGraw-Hill Education; 2016. pp. 1137-1175

[4] Sajid MS, Khawaja AH, Sains P, Singh KK, Baig MK. A systematic review comparing laparoscopic vs open adhesiolysis in patients with adhesional small bowel obstruction. American Journal of Surgery. 2016;**212**(1):138-150

[5] Pezzoli A, Maimone A, Fusetti N, et al. Gallstone ileus treated with non-surgical conservative methods: A case report. Journal of Medical Case Reports. 2015;**9**:15. DOI: 10.1186/1752-1947-9-15

[6] Neri V. Management of intestinal obstruction. In: Garbuzenko DV, editor. Actual Problems of Emergency Abdominal Surgery. IntechOpen; 2016. DOI: 10.5772/63156

[7] Kocaay AF, Çelik SU, Eker T, Çetinkaya ÖA, Genç V. Intraperitoneal adhesions: Pathogenesis, clinical significance, and prevention strategies. The Medical Bulletin of Sisli Etfal Hospital. 2015;**49**(4):231-237

[8] Shelton BK. Intestinal obstruction. AACN Clinical Issues. 1999;**10**(4):478-491

[9] Al Gharbi AF, Al Shammari MSA, Al Marshadi JAA, Al Awad MN, Al Qufayi AA, Al Shaya HK, et al. The clinical presentations and patterns of management of bowel obstruction in northern Saudi Arabia. Surgical Science. 2018;**9**:174-181

[10] Hussain J, Alrashed AM, Alkhadher T, Wood S, Behbehani AD, Termos S. Gall stone ileus: Unfamiliar cause of bowel obstruction. Case report and literature review. International Journal of Surgery Case Reports. 2018;**49**:44-50

[11] Bevan PG. Intestinal obstruction. British Medical Journal. 1968;**1**(5593):687-690

[12] Hollerweger A, Wüstner M, Dirks K. Bowel obstruction: Sonographic evaluation. Ultraschall In Der Medizin. 2015;**36**(3):216-235; quiz 236-8

[13] Shiomi H, Shimizu T, Endo Y, et al. Relations among circulating monocytes, dendritic cells, and bacterial translocation in patients with intestinal obstruction. World Journal of Surgery. 2007;**31**:1806-1812

[14] Vilz TO, Stoffels B, Strassburg C, Schild HH, Kalff JC. Ileus in adults. Deutsches Ärzteblatt International. 2017;**114**(29-30):508-518. DOI: 10.3238/arztebl.2017.0508

[15] Hwabejire JO, Tran DD, Fullum TM. Non-operative management of adhesive small bowel obstruction: Should there be a time limit after which surgery is performed? American Journal of Surgery. 2018;**215**(6):1068-1070

[16] Zhu W. Prevention and management of intestinal obstruction after gastrointestinal surgery. Zhonghua Wei Chang Wai Ke Za Zhi. 2016;**19**(4):376-378

[17] Hayden GE, Sprouse KL. Bowel obstruction and hernia. Emergency Medicine Clinics of North America. 2011;**29**(2):319-345

[18] Aktürk OM, Aktürk Y, Aydoğan İ. Diagnosis and treatment of small intestines obstruction. Bozok Medical Journal. 2015;**5**(3):51-54

[19] Altınel M, Akıncı S. Postoperative care in urologic laparoscopic surgery. Turkish Urology Seminars. 2010;**1**:147-152

[20] Dağistanli S, Kalaycı MU, Kara Y. Evaluation of ERAS protocol in general surgery. Istanbul Kanuni Sultan Süleyman Medical Journal. 2018;**10**(suppl):9-20

[21] Ersoy E, Gündoğdu H. Enhanced recovery after surgery. Turkish Journal of Surgery. 2007;**23**(1):035040

[22] Güllüoglu BM, Akın ML, Barlas A, Erenoğlu C, Aktan AÖ, Batkın A. Is nasogastric decompression mandatory after colon and rectum surgery? A prospective randomized study. Turkish Journal of Surgery. 2000;**16**(4): 245-253

[23] Çilingir D, Şahin UC. Patient-controlled analgesia in surgical patient. Journal of Hacettepe University Faculty of Nursing. 2016;**3**(3):56-69

[24] Şenyüz KY, Koçaşli S. Multimodal analgesy and nursing approach in postoperative pain. Sağ Aka Derg. 2017;**4**(2):90-95

[25] Dumlu EG, Bozkurt B, Tokaç M, Kiyak G, Özkardeş AB, Yalçın S, et al. Malnutrition and nutrition supplementation in surgical patients. Ankara Medical Journal. 2013;**13**(1):33-39

[26] Foster NM, McGory ML, Zingmond DS, Ko CY. Small bowel obstruction: A population-based appraisal. Journal of the American College of Surgeons. 2006;**203**(2):170-176

[27] Schraufnagel D, Rajaee S, Millham FH. How many sunsets? Timing of surgery in adhesive small bowel obstruction: A study of the nationwide inpatient sample. Journal of Trauma and Acute Care Surgery. 2013;**74**(1):181-187

[28] Fazel MZ, Jamieson RW, Watson CJ. Long-term follow-up of the use of the Jones' intestinal tube in adhesive small bowel obstruction. Annals of the Royal College of Surgeons of England. 2009;**91**(1):50-54

[29] Ozturk E, van Iersel M, Stommel MM, et al. Small bowel obstruction in the elderly: A plea for comprehensive acute geriatric care. World Journal of Emergency Surgery : WJES. 2018;**13**:48

[30] Karabulut M, Gönenç M, İslim F, Kalaycı MU, Kapan S, Turhan AN, et al. Acute mechanical bowel obstruction: A 5-year experience in a training and research hospital. Turkish Journal of Surgery. 2011;**27**(1):010-014

[31] Ko YT, Lim JH, Lee DH, et al. Small bowel obstruction: Sonographic evaluation. Radiology. 1993;**188**:649-653

[32] Suri S, Gupta S, Sudhakar PJ, et al. Comparative evaluation of plain films, ultrasound and CT in the diagnosis of intestinal obstruction. Acta Radiologica. 1999;**40**:422

[33] Mallo RD, Salem R, Lalani T, et al. Computed tomography diagnosis of ischemia and complete obstruction in small bowel obstruction: A systematic review. Journal of Gastrointestinal Surgery. 2005;**9**:690-694

[34] Maglinte DDT, Heitkamp DE, Howard TJ, Kelvin FM, Lappas JC. Current concepts in imaging of small bowel obstruction. Radiologic Clinics of North America. 2003;**41**:263-283

[35] Targownik LE, Spiegel BM, Sack J, et al. Colonic stent vs. emergency surgery for management of acute left-sided malignant colonic obstruction: A decision analysis. Gastrointestinal Endoscopy. 2004;**60**:865-874

[36] Vitale MA, Villotti G, D'Alba L, et al. Preoperative colonoscopy after self-expandable metallic stent placement in patients with acute neoplastic colon obstruction. Gastrointestinal Endoscopy. 2006;**63**:814-819

[37] Soto S, Lopez-Roses L, Gonzalez-Ramirez A, et al. Endoscopic treatment of acute colorectal obstruction with selfexpandable metallic stents: Experience in a community hospital. Surgical Endoscopy. 2006;**20**:1072-1076

[38] Connolly MM, Unti JA, Nora PF. Bowel obstruction in pregnancy. The Surgical Clinics of North America. 1995;**75**(1):101-113. DOI: 10.1016/s0039-6109(16)46537-0

[39] Polat Düzdün A, Özmen M, Coşkun F. Intestinal obstruction in pregnancy: A review. Turkiye Klinikleri J Gynecol Obst. 2003;**13**(6):476-482

[40] Lopez Carral JM, Esen UI, Chandrashekar MV, Rogers IM, Olajide F. Volvulus of the right colon in pregnancy. International Journal of Clinical Practice. 1998;**52**(4):270-271

Section 4

Infections and Recovery

Chapter 6

Invasive Aspergillosis in Transplant Recipients

Marta Wróblewska, Beata Sulik-Tyszka, Wojciech Figiel, Grzegorz Niewiński and Krzysztof Zieniewicz

Abstract

Patients with hematological malignancies and recipients of allogeneic hematopoietic stem cell transplantation (allo-HSCT) as well as solid organ transplant recipients are the groups of patients with the highest risk of invasive fungal infections (IFI). Neutropenia, lymphopenia, chemotherapy of malignancies, radiation therapy, immunosuppressive therapy, administration of glucocorticosteroids, use of central venous catheters, dialysis therapy, liver and kidney failure, and diabetes are diseases and medical conditions which foster invasive fungal infections. In recent years, it has been observed that the most common etiological agents of these infections are yeast-like fungi of the genus Candida, and the second most common is moulds *Aspergillus* spp. Antifungal agent recommended for therapy of IFI caused by *Aspergillus* is voriconazole, according to the present guidelines. A combined therapy using voriconazole and caspofungin may not be effective. According to numerous publications, in case of infections caused by strains resistant to voriconazole, a therapeutic success is possible after a switch to the liposomal form of amphotericin B. Due to nonspecific clinical symptoms of IFI caused by *Aspergillus* spp., histopathological as well as mycological and serological tests, echocardiographic examination, magnetic resonance imaging (MRI) and computer tomography (CT) may contribute to an early and reliable diagnosis of invasive aspergillosis.

Keywords: *Aspergillus fumigatus*, invasive fungal infection, risk factors, antifungal therapy

1. Introduction

Transplant recipients constitute a group of patients who are immunocompromised. Among them, hematopoietic stem cell transplant (HSCT) recipients suffer from the most severe immunosuppression, which may be prolonged. Many risk factors make these patients prone to fungal infections caused by yeast-like fungi or molds.

Filamentous fungi of the genus *Aspergillus* may cause many clinical forms of the disease in immunocompromised patients (including HSCT recipients and solid organ transplant recipients), but increasingly also in patients undergoing intensive care or even without any immune deficiencies [1]. Aspergillosis usually results from inhalation of spores, affecting primarily the respiratory system [1–3]. Humans are exposed daily to massive numbers of fungal spores; however, usually they are eliminated by various pulmonary defense mechanisms, for example, mucociliary function [1, 2]. With progress in molecular diagnostic methods, particularly next-generation sequencing (NGS) techniques, we have learned that molds and yeast-like fungi are present in the respiratory tract, even in healthy individuals [4]. Similar to microbiota composition in other parts of the body, the lung mycobiota also comprises numerous fungal species, which become less diverse in many diseases [4].

Aspergillosis may present in different forms, such as invasive aspergillosis (IA), allergic aspergillosis, chronic pulmonary aspergillosis, and as superficial disease in various anatomical locations (keratitis, otomycosis, and wound infections) [1, 4–6]. Allergic aspergillosis may present as allergic bronchopulmonary aspergillosis (ABPA) and allergic fungal rhinosinusitis (AFRS) [7].

Invasive aspergillosis is further divided into invasive pulmonary aspergillosis (IPA), sinusitis caused by *Aspergillus* spp., disseminated aspergillosis, and several types of invasive aspergillosis with the involvement of single organs [5, 6]. In transplant recipients and other immunocompromised patients, the most common clinical form of aspergillosis is invasive pulmonary aspergillosis, which untreated or unsuccessfully treated can lead to systemic dissemination to other organs and systems, for example, brain, heart, or the bones [1, 2]. In contrast, paranasal sinuses, larynx, eyes, ears, and the oral cavity are often involved in primary aspergillosis [2].

Invasive aspergillosis is the most common mold infection, particularly among immunocompromised patients. Patients subjected to allogeneic hematopoietic stem cell transplantation (alloHSCT) constitute a group of patients with the highest risk of systemic fungal infections, caused by both *Candida* spp., as well as *Aspergillus* spp. [5, 6]. Factors predisposing to the invasive aspergillosis are prolonged neutropenia (<500/μl for >10 days) and lymphopenia (mainly affecting CD4+ cells) [5, 8–12]. Frequency of invasive infections caused by *Aspergillus* spp. is on the increase in patients undergoing chemo- and/or radiotherapy, treated with corticosteroids or immunosuppressive agents, as well as in patients with acquired immune deficiency syndrome (AIDS) or congenital deficiencies of the immune system, such as chronic granulomatous disease [1, 8, 10, 12–14]. Patients at the extremes of age (>60 and neonates), persons with chronic malnutrition, and individuals on total parenteral nutrition have fungal infections more often than patients in other groups [8, 10, 13]. Surgical procedures, particularly thoracic or abdominal surgery and solid organ transplantation, and the use of central venous catheters or dialysis catheters are linked to endogenous and exogenous infections, including those caused by *Aspergillus* spp. [1, 5, 6, 8–11]. Underlying diseases, such as diabetes, kidney, and/or liver failure, and chronic obstructive pulmonary disease (COPD) also predispose to invasive fungal infections [1, 8].

2. Etiology of invasive aspergillosis

Aspergillosis is caused by opportunistic molds of the genus *Aspergillus*, which contains more than 300 species; however, only relatively few of them are known to cause human diseases [12]. These fungi are ubiquitous in soil, plants, and decaying organic debris, as well as in household dust and building materials [1]. Hospitalized immunocompromised patients are at risk of aspergillosis during construction or renovation works at the hospital. Fungi *Aspergillus* spp. (like other molds), produce conidia that are easily aerosolized [12]. Inhaled conidia colonize the respiratory system of the host in whom—depending on the degree of immunosuppression—various clinical forms of aspergillosis may develop. Rarely, aspergillosis results from ingestion of the spores or their direct inoculation into the wounds [12].

The most common etiological agent of invasive aspergillosis with a high morality is *A. fumigatus*, responsible for the majority (up to 90%) of cases in humans [1, 12, 15–19]. It is followed by *A. flavus*, which causes up to 10% of cases of bronchoalveolar aspergillosis [18]. This species also is responsible for most cases of aspergillosis with sinus and skin involvement [1]. It appears that *A. flavus* survives better than other *Aspergillus* spp. in a dry and hot climate; therefore, it is mainly isolated in Asia, Middle East, and Africa [17]. Other species of the genus *Aspergillus*, such as *A. niger*, *A. nidulans*, *A. terreus*, *A. versicolor*, *A. calidoustus*, and *A. ustus* cause invasive infections less frequently; however, they are of importance in immunocompromised patients [12, 18, 20, 21]. Strains of *A. niger* colonize the respiratory tract and are etiological agents of most cases of external otitis [1]. According to the Prospective Antifungal Therapy Alliance® (PATH Alliance ®) registry, in a cohort study of 960 cases of proven/probable IA, *A. fumigatus* (72.6%) was the most predominant species, followed by *A. flavus* (9.9%), *A. niger* (8.7%), and *A. terreus* (4.3%) [12]. Recently, an increasing frequency of infections caused by environmental species of *Aspergillus* (of unknown significance in medicine) is being reported [21].

Apart from *Aspergillus* species other than *A. fumigatus*, recently attention is being focused on the strains classified in the section Fumigati (*A. fumigatus* complex), for example, *Neosartorya udagawae* (*A. udagawae*) [18, 22]. They may cause similar diseases as *A. fumigatus sensu stricto*; however, duration of illness may be prolonged (even sevenfold) [22]. It appears that actual prevalence of these cases may be underestimated, as these strains are often misidentified because they cannot be distinguished from *A. fumigatus sensu stricto* by conventional morphological tests [18]. Moreover, the outcome of treatment of these infections may be unfavorable, as strains belonging to *A. fumigatus*-related species (the section Fumigati) often show some level of intrinsic resistance to azoles and other antifungal drugs, with the minimum inhibitory concentrations (MICs) of various antifungals for these isolates higher than those for *A. fumigatus*, which is usually susceptible to azoles [22]. However, in a recent multicenter prospective study, the rate of azole resistance among *A. fumigatus* isolates was relatively high—3.2%, out of which 78% were *A. fumigatus sensu stricto* with a mutation of the *cyp51A* gene, while the remaining 22% were the related species (*A. lentulus*, *A. thermomutatus*, and *A. udagawae*) [23].

In clinical practice *A. lentulus*, *A. udagawae*, *A. viridinutans*, and *A. thermomutatus* (*Neosartorya pseudofischeri*), *A. novofumigatus* and *A. hiratsukae* have been linked etiologically to such refractory cases of IA [18]. These *A. fumigatus* complex strains are characterized by lower virulence ascribed to a lower thermotolerance and different profiles of secondary metabolites with decreased production of mycotoxins, such as gliotoxin [18]. Definitive identification of these cryptic species requires specific sequencing analyses of the beta-tubulin or calmodulin genes, which are not readily available. Clinical microbiologists should, therefore, be aware of such cryptic species of *Aspergillus* and the methods of their differentiation from *A. fumigatus*—defect in sporulation, unusual susceptibility profile to antifungals, as well as multiplex PCR assays and matrix-assisted laser desorption ionization time-of-flight mass spectrometry (MALDI-TOF MS) technique [18].

3. Clinical forms of invasive aspergillosis

Molds of the genus *Aspergillus* may cause a wide variety of clinical entities, ranging from asymptomatic colonization, allergic bronchopulmonary aspergillosis, and chronic pulmonary aspergillosis to severe (even fulminant) invasive infections in almost every organ or system in the body of the host, including (but not limited to) the lungs, heart, central nervous system, and the sinuses [5, 18, 19, 24]. The most common clinical form of invasive diseases caused by *Aspergillus* spp. is pulmonary aspergillosis, which in about 50% of cases spreads to other anatomical locations, including the brain, liver, kidneys, endocardium, bones, and gastrointestinal tract [8, 10, 13, 19, 25]. Aspergillosis may also affect the paranasal sinuses, the ear, or the eyeball [13].

The spectrum of aspergillosis is determined by the host's immune status (particularly severe and prolonged neutropenia) and the virulence of *Aspergillus* strain causing the infection [5, 6, 12, 13]. In immunocompetent persons, molds of the genus *Aspergillus* mainly cause allergic symptoms and chronic pulmonary aspergillosis, without invasion and destruction of the host's tissues [12]. In the chronic pulmonary aspergillosis, usually a preexisting pulmonary condition is observed, such as preformed cavity in the lung (resulting from tuberculosis, sarcoidosis, or other necrotising process), in which an aspergilloma (or a fungus ball) is being formed (chronic cavitary pulmonary aspergillosis) [12]. Allergic bronchopulmonary aspergillosis (ABPA) is a disease that arises from a hypersensitivity reaction to *Aspergillus* antigens and most often develops in patients who have asthma, atopy, or cystic fibrosis [8, 12, 26]. Another form of aspergillosis, characterized by a local invasion of the lung parenchyma; however, without invasion or dissemination to other organs, is called subacute invasive aspergillosis (or chronic necrotizing pulmonary aspergillosis) [12].

Invasive aspergillosis is a life-threatening infection and a major cause of death in immunocompromised patients, particularly hematopoietic stem cell transplant recipients, but may be fatal even in immunocompetent individuals, with the death rate of 40% for pulmonary disease, 90% for disseminated disease, and practically 100% for disseminated disease with the central nervous system (CNS) involvement [1, 19]. According to the literature, invasive aspergillosis occurs in 1–15% of the solid organ transplant recipients, in whom mortality rates due to this disease range from 65 to 92% [1]. However, currently these indices improve in these patients due to advances in immunosuppressive regimens and transplantation practices, as well as frequent use of antifungal prophylaxis.

Recent reports indicate that invasive aspergillosis is being increasingly diagnosed in patients without above-mentioned severe neutropenia—particularly in the lung transplant recipients, patients hospitalized in the intensive care unit or treated with corticosteroids [9, 11, 27]. Also, individuals with chronic obstructive pulmonary disease (COPD), liver failure, and other underlying diseases are listed in this group [8, 11, 20]. It has been reported that in ICU patients with invasive pulmonary aspergillosis 40–80% of them do not have any malignancy or other classical risk factors for this infection [8, 20]. Moreover, in contrast to patients with neutropenia, in ICU patients the symptoms of aspergillosis are atypical; therefore the diagnosis of this infection may be delayed or omitted, according to the autopsy studies [11, 15, 28]. Tejerina et al. showed that among 893 deceased patients, previously treated in ICU, only 40% (10 out of 25) had invasive aspergillosis diagnosed *ante mortem* [11]. Problems with proper diagnosis of invasive asergillosis, and therefore a delay in administration of effective antifungal therapy, are undoubtfully linked to a high mortality rate in this group of patients (30–40%), which may even exceed 90% despite lack of severe immunosuppression in these individuals [15, 27, 29].

3.1 Aspergillosis of the oral cavity and the upper respiratory tract

As mentioned earlier, aspergillosis affects mainly the lungs; however it may also be diagnosed in the upper respiratory tract and the oral cavity [2, 30]. Orofacial aspergillosis is relatively common in oncohematological patients undergoing chemotherapy [2].

Aspergillosis of the larynx is very rare, with only a few cases reported in the literature [31]. Usually, it is secondary form of this disease, while primary aspergillosis of the larynx is even rarer. Risk factors for aspergillosis of the larynx comprise the use of inhaled or systemic steroids, prolonged antibiotic therapy, and underlying immunosuppression [31]. It should be emphasized that these lesions may mimic malignancy or a premalignant condition, while proper diagnosis and administration of antifungal therapy, as well as elimination of the risk factors (if possible), are effective in the elimination of this condition [31].

It also appears that chronic tonsillitis may be caused by *Aspergillus* spp. In a study of 75 symptomatic children who underwent a tonsillectomy, in 9 (12%) of them *Aspergillus* was detected on histological examination of the removed tonsils [30].

Aspergillus spores may be deposited in the oral cavity upon inhalation or during dental procedures, for example, tooth extraction [3]. The fungus may then spread further into the sinuses as odontogenic infection [32, 33]. The infection may also become established in the oral cavity itself.

In oral aspergillosis, the lesions are usually located on the palate or posterior tongue [2]. They are yellow or black, with a necrotic ulcerated base. The hyphal elements of *Aspergillus* fungus may invade the oral mucosa through the release of various toxins, such as proteases, phospholipases, hemolysins, gliotoxin, aflatoxin, phthioic acid, and many others. Subsequently, they penetrate the blood vessels, producing thrombosis, infarction and necrosis, and then systemic spread follows [2].

3.2 Aspergillosis of the nose and paranasal sinuses

Paranasal sinuses may be colonized or infected by fungi, while infection can be invasive (acute or chronic) or noninvasive (allergic sinusitis and aspergilloma) [18]. In invasive aspergillosis of the sinuses, there are rapid (within a few days) destructions of the sinuses, the nasal cavity, and the adjacent structures, such as the orbit and the brain [18]. *Aspergillus* spp. may also cause allergic *Aspergillus* sinusitis (AAS), which results from a hypersensitivity reaction to the presence of the fungus in the sinus [26]. The hallmark of AAS is demonstration of fungal elements in the material obtained from the sinus [26].

It is estimated, that fungal sinusitis constitutes 6–9% of all cases of rhinosinusitis. Among fungi causing sinusitis, the most common is *Aspergillus* spp. [18]. Aspergillosis of the paranasal sinus should be suspected in patients with refractory or recurrent sinusitis. Apart from the sinuses, aspergillosis may also affect the nasal cavity, from which the infection can spread to the CNS (rhinocerebral aspergillosis).

The maxillary sinus is more often affected than other paranasal sinuses. However, it is frequently misdiagnosed, even as malignancy [3, 18, 34]. Untreated infection may spread to the other structures in the head [35]. Invasive aspergillosis of the maxillary sinus should be considered in patients with maxillary sinusitis which does not respond to standard therapy with antibiotics, even in immunocompetent patients [3].

From the paranasal sinuses, *Aspergillus* infection may spread locally into the vasculature and the brain, leading to cavernous sinus thrombosis and a variety of central nervous system manifestations and to other locations, for example, the orbit [36]. In these cases, computed tomography (CT) or magnetic resonance imaging (MRI) and biopsy of any lesion located in the sinuses or the nasal cavity in high-risk patients is mandatory [19]. Intracranial and intraorbital extension decreases the survival rate of these patients [3].

Factors which predispose immunocompetent individuals to fungal infections in the sinuses include polyps and blocked drainage of secretions [3]. Additional risk factors for fungal sinusitis, including *Aspergillus*, are reported in immunocompromised patients and individuals with various underlying diseases, such as neutropenia, immunosuppressive therapy, corticosteroids, uncontrolled diabetes mellitus, trauma, burns, and radiation therapy [3]. In these patients, particularly with hematological malignancies and in transplant recipients, *Aspergillus* may cause an invasive infection as aggressive in its clinical course as those caused by *Zygomycetes* [19]. Invasive fungal sinusitis is potentially fatal, with an extremely high mortality rate, particularly in immunocompromised patients [3]. Therefore invasive aspergillosis of the paranasal sinuses has to be recognized and treated to avoid significant mortality in immunocompromised patients, particularly in transplant recipients [3]. It should be suspected in cases of purulent rhinosinusitis not responding to repeated courses of antibiotics, and on the basis of radiological features.

Therapy of fungal sinusitis depends on its clinical form. In cases of *Aspergillus* fungal ball of the paranasal sinuses, surgical removal alone can be sufficient [5, 6]. Enlargement of the sinus opening may be needed to improve drainage and prevent further recurrence of sinusitis [5, 6]. In invasive aspergillosis apart from surgery, also systemic antifugal therapy is recommended.

3.3 Aspergillosis of the lower respiratory tract

Within the lower respiratory tract, *Aspergillus* infection may affect the larynx, trachea, and bronchi (tracheobronchitis), as well as lung parenchyma (pulmonary aspergillosis). In rare cases, *Aspergillus* pleuritis has been reported [19].

The lungs are affected in up to 92% of all cases of invasive aspergillosis [19]. Invasive pulmonary aspergillosis is a clinical entity characterized by invasion of the fungal hyphae into the blood vessels (angioinvasion), which subsequent hemoptysis. Other symptoms comprise nonproductive cough, pleuritic pain, low-grade fever, and dyspnea [19]. However, in the early stages of the disease, both clinical symptoms and radiological findings may be nonspecific, so proper diagnosis and treatment may be delayed, resulting in increased mortality in this group of patients.

The frequency of invasive pulmonary aspergillosis has significantly increased in recent years due to a growing number of immunocompromised patients [8, 37]. This clinical entity most often occurs in patients with different forms of immunosuppression, for example, hematological malignancies, profound and prolonged neutropenia, or corticosteroid therapy, as well as organ transplantation, autoimmune and inflammatory conditions, in critically ill patients, and those with chronic obstructive pulmonary disease (COPD) [8, 37]. In about 50% of patients with invasive pulmonary aspergillosis, the infection spreads to other anatomical sites, such as the brain, liver, kidneys, or the gastrointestinal tract [8, 10, 13, 19, 25].

An uncommon clinical form of IA is an isolated invasive *Aspergillus* tracheobronchitis (iIATB), in which fungal infection is limited predominantly or entirely to the tracheobronchial tree [19, 38]. It has been mainly reported in lung- and heart-lung transplant recipients. Wu et al. reviewed 19 cases of this disease and concluded that iIATB occurs in moderately or nonimmunocompromised patients with impaired airway structures or defense functions and it may be an early period of invasive pulmonary aspergillosis [38]. Early diagnosis and effective antifungal treatment were linked to a favorable prognosis; however, 5 out of 19 (26.3%) patients died.

Other forms of *Aspergillus* infection of the lungs comprise chronic necrotizing aspergillosis, which is described in patients with chronic lung disease or low degree immunodeficiency as a locally invasive disease, as well as aspergilloma usually found in individuals with previously formed cavities in the lungs [8, 12].

As mentioned earlier, symptoms of the pulmonary disease may result not from actual infection, but allergic reaction of the host to the presence of *Aspergillus* in the bronchial tree—allergic brochopulmonary aspergillosis (ABPA) [12, 26].

This immunologically mediated disease occurs predominantly in patients with asthma, atopy, and cystic fibrosis (CF) [8, 12, 26].

3.4 Aspergillosis of the central nervous system

Aspergillosis of the brain (cerebral aspergillosis) is usually a part of the disseminated disease after hematogenous spread of infection from the lungs, but rarely it may represent an isolated disease of the central nervous system (CNS) [19]. It is reported in 10–15% of patients with invasive pulmonary aspergillosis [39]. The most common risk factors comprise neutropenia and other forms of immunosuppression and transplantation surgery [19]. Cerebral aspergillosis usually presents as a single or multiple brain abscess, also as cerebral vasculitis and cerebral infarcts, while meningitis is rare [19]. Brain abscesses are common in HSCT recipients, while relatively rare in solid organ transplant (SOT) recipients [40, 41]. CT and MRI are recommended in patients in whom cerebral aspergillosis is suspected [42]. Among all types of IA, brain aspergillosis has the worst prognosis, with mortality rate usually exceeding 90% (up to 100%), however early and proper treatment improves the prognosis in these patients and significantly increases their survival rates [19].

Aspergillosis of the CNS may also present as rhinocerebral aspergillosis, particularly in patients with underlying malignancies and neutropenia, HSCT recipients, and patients with diabetic ketoacidosis [37]. Symptoms usually comprise fever, nasal or sinus congestion or pain, nasal discharge, unilateral facial swelling, and headaches [37]. Necrotic lesions may be seen on the hard palate and in the nasal cavity. The spread of infection may lead to ophthalmic complications, such as ptosis, proptosis, and vision disturbances [37].

3.5 Invasive cardiac aspergillosis

Invasive cardiac aspergillosis may present as endocarditis, myocarditis, pericarditis, mediastinitis, septic thrombophlebitis, and infections of aortic grafts—also in transplant recipients [5, 6, 43, 44].

Endocarditis caused by *Aspergillus* spp. is a severe form of fungal endocarditis [45, 46]. The mortality rate is high and surgery is usually required [19, 45–47]. It is very rare, but in recent years, the incidence of this form of aspergillosis is increasing, due to a rise in the frequency of its risk factors—the use of invasive procedures involving the heart, cardiac surgery with replacement of the heart valves, implantation of cardiac devices, organ transplantation, drug abuse, or administration of immunosuppressive therapy [19, 45]. Pierrotti and Baddour analyzed mold-related endocarditis in 3939 patients (the majority of cases were caused by *Aspergillus* spp.) and found the following risk factors: underlying cardiac abnormalities (41%), prosthetic heart valves (39%), malignancy (18%), solid-organ transplantation (18%), and bone marrow transplantation (18%) [47]. In a study by Paterson et al., 26% of cases of infective endocarditis occurring within a month of solid organ transplantation were caused by *Aspergillus* [48]. Woods et al. found that the most common predisposing factors for *Aspergillus* endocarditis in 29 patients were corticosteroid therapy (55%), prolonged antibiotic treatment (31%), hematological malignancy (28%), and chemotherapy and cytotoxic therapy (28%) [49].

In the course of *Aspergillus* endocarditis, mitral and bicuspid valves (native or prosthetic) are most often affected [19, 46, 50, 51]. Fungal vegetations may be formed on the heart valves, which subsequently may cause embolism blocking the arteries. Gumbo et al. reported that vegetations were revealed on the heart valves in 78% of the cases in which echocardiography was performed, while embolic episodes were seen in 69% of patients with *Aspergillus* endocarditis, and a new or changing heart murmur—in 41% of them [52]. In a recently published study, Meshaal et al. showed that aortic abscess or pseudoaneurysm was one of the strong predictors of *Aspergillus* endocarditis [45]. However, it should be noted that *Aspergillus* endocarditis may be difficult to diagnose because blood cultures are usually negative, while fever is absent in 26% of patients with this disease [19, 45]. *Aspergillus* endocarditis should, therefore, be suspected in patients with underlying immunosuppression, hematological malignancies, recent cardiothoracic surgery, intravenous drug use, systemic or pulmonary emboli with negative blood cultures, and vegetation on echocardiography [24]. Diagnosis should be confirmed by histology and mycological culture of tissue or vegetation samples [24]. Delayed or erroneous diagnosis of *Aspergillus* endocarditis contributes to incorrect management of patients. Early surgical replacement of an infected valve and prolonged administration of antifungal therapy (which may be lifelong) are recommended to prevent embolic complications, valvular decompensation, and further spread of the infection [5, 6, 24, 43, 44].

Heart muscle may be affected by *Aspergillus* infection in the form of myocarditis or cardiomyopathy [53, 54]. This form of disease usually results from hematogenous spread of infection and is characterized by the presence of abscesses. Pericarditis caused by *Aspergillus* spp. has been described, also in transplant recipients [43, 55].

3.6 Ocular aspergillosis

Aspergillosis of the eye may take a form of fungal keratitis, endophthalmitis, or invasive aspergillosis of the orbit. All structures of the eyeball may be affected—eyelids, conjunctivae, lacrimal apparatus, cornea, sclera, or uvea. *Aspergillus* dacryocystitis is a rare complication of aspergillosis of the paranasal sinuses [56]. Clinicians must be aware that the clinical course of ocular aspergillosis may range from asymptomatic infection or slowly developing disease to rapidly progressive infection, with a fulminant course and fatal outcome [56].

Fungal keratitis often presents as a corneal ulcer, which results from mechanical injury of the cornea, with subsequent necrosis. In a recent study, Manikandan et al. examined a total of 500 corneal scrapings, collected from patients in whom mycotic keratitis was suspected, out of which 68 (13.6%) were positive for *Aspergillus* spp. [57].

Endophthalmitis may be a complication of surgical procedures or may result from hematogenous spread from other sites of infection. Endogenous *Aspergillus* endophthalmitis is mainly reported in severely immunocompromised patients, transplant organ recipients, patients after heart valve replacement, and in oncohematological patients [58–60].

Orbital invasive aspergillosis is a rare infection, which most often results from dissemination of the infection from the nose or paranasal sinuses. It may take an acute or chronic form. This form of IA usually presents with a severe orbital pain, paralysis of the oculomotor nerve and visual impairment. Ophthalmic complications, such as ptosis, proptosis, and vision disturbances may result from the spread of infection in rhinocerebral aspergillosis [37].

3.7 Aspergillosis of the genitourinary tract

Aspergillosis of the urinary tract is relatively rare. In immunocompromised patients, such as kidney transplant recipients, frequency of this form of aspergillosis amounts to only 0.5–2.2%, but is fatal in >88% of patients [61]. Urinary tract aspergillosis may also be a complication of surgical procedures, such as lithotripsy, urinary tract instrumentation, or ureteric stenting, particularly in immunocompromised patients [62–65]. Renal aspergillosis is being occasionally reported with obstruction of one or both ureters [19]. Localized aspergillosis of the renal graft was reported in a child 5 months after kidney transplantation [61]. A case of urinary tract aspergillosis presenting as an aspergilloma of the urinary bladder has also been described [66].

Aspergillosis of the genital tract has been rarely reported [67–69]. In women, it may give the symptoms resembling a pelvic inflammatory disease.

3.8 Other clinical forms of aspergillosis

Other clinical forms of aspergillosis—apart from above-mentioned—are very rare and comprise gastrointestinal aspergillosis, cutaneous aspergillosis, *Aspergillus* peritonitis, osteomyelitis, and septic arthritis, as well as *Aspergillus* ear infections [5, 6, 19, 37].

Gastrointestinal aspergillosis is mainly reported in patients who are transplant recipients or severely malnourished [37]. It results from ingestion of *Aspergillus* spp. spores. The most commonly involved sites are the stomach, colon, and ileum.

Cutaneous aspergillosis is classified as primary or secondary [37]. Primary form of the disease is usually reported in patients with burn wounds or surgical wounds. This clinical entity is caused by direct inoculation of the fungus or its spores into the injured skin [37]. Primary cutaneous aspergillosis has been linked to leukemic patients, neonates, transplant recipients, as well as the use of occlusive dressings or permanent intravenous catheters [19]. Secondary cutaneous aspergillosis results from hematogenous spread of the fungus and therefore represents a disseminated form of *Aspergillus* infection. It may present as nodules or extensive necrotic lesions [19]. The mortality rate may be high.

Aspergillus peritonitis is seen in patients undergoing peritoneal dialysis [19]. It may be complicated by hemorrhage, perforation, or infarction.

Aspergillus ear infections may present as noninvasive otitis externa (otomycosis) or invasive aspergillosis of the ear. Examples of other forms of invasive aspergillosis comprise vertebral osteomyelitis (resulting from hematogenous spread, by contiguity or from direct inoculation), septic arthritis, cholangitis, and prosthetic vascular graft rejection [19].

Disseminated aspergillosis if defined as the involvement of at least two noncontiguous sites in the body, mainly in transplant recipients [19]. Disseminated disease has been reported in 9–36% of kidney transplant recipients, 15–20% of lung transplant recipients, 20–35% of heart transplant recipients, and 50–60% of liver transplant recipients with invasive aspergillosis [70].

4. Aspergillosis in transplant recipients

In patients with immune deficiencies and other risk factors, invasive aspergillosis (IA) is a life-threatening infection caused by the opportunistic molds of the genus *Aspergillus*, most often by *A. fumigatus* [5, 6, 14, 70, 71]. A cohort study of 960 cases of probable or proven IA reported in the Prospective Antifungal Therapy Alliance (PATH Alliance) registry, indicated that 48.3% of patients had hematologic malignancy, 29.2% were SOT recipients, 27.9% were HSCT recipients, and 33.8% were neutropenic [12]. In these patients, the most common clinical forms of IA are invasive pulmonary aspergillosis (IPA) and rhinocerebral aspergillosis [12].

In transplant recipients, particularly in hematopoietic stem cell transplant (HSCT) recipients who are severely immunocompromised, invasive aspergillosis is not only more common than in other groups of patients, but is also characterized by much more severe and rapidly progressive clinical course, and much higher mortality [12, 72].

Although prognosis has improved in recent years, IA still remains a significant post-transplant complication in solid organ transplant (SOT) recipients [43, 44]. It occurs in up to 30% of SOT recipients. Although in recent years the mortality rate in transplant recipients decreased from 65–92% to 22%, still an estimated 9.3–16.9% of all deaths in transplant recipients in the first year after transplantation can be attributed to IA [44].

The incidence of IA differs between different populations of transplant recipients, and unique risk factors for *Aspergillus* infections have been identified for various types of organ transplant recipients [43, 44]. However, regardless of the type of transplantation a major risk factor for the development of IA in SOT recipients is the net state of immunosuppression including the intensity of administered immunosuppressive therapy [44].

Regarding the risk of invasive fungal infections (particularly IA) in transplant recipients, at present routine antifungal prophylaxis or preemptive therapy is recommended in HSCT recipients with prolonged neutropenia or graft-versus-host disease (GVHD), and in lung transplant recipients, while targeted prophylaxis should be considered in liver and heart transplant recipients [5, 6, 44, 71].

4.1 Hematopoietic stem cell transplant (HSCT) recipients

Invasive aspergillosis remains a major complication following allogeneic HSCT (alloHSCT) [73]. The burden of IA has increased significantly in the last 30 years as a result of the increased number of patients undergoing immunosuppressive therapy for hematological malignancies and HSCT [14]. It is estimated that IA is a leading cause of fatal outcomes in HSCT patients, accounting for 10% of all deaths in this group of patients [14].

In the recipients of alloHSCT, IA can occur during the neutropenic pre-engraftment phase (early IA) or during the post-engraftment period (late IA) [14]. Although IA remains an important complication after allogeneic transplantation, regardless of the type of conditioning regimen, early IA is more common in patients undergoing myeloablative transplantation due to extensive chemotherapy and radiation used to destroy the native bone marrow, and prolonged neutropenia which results from this treatment [14, 74]. On the other hand, non-myeloablative HSCT comprises a shorter neutropenic period and therefore, a decrease in the incidence of early IA. However, a higher risk of GVHD in this group of patients and the therapies given for this condition caused a shift to late IA, diagnosed increasingly during the post-engraftment period [14]. It should be noted that the risk period for late IA, associated with GVHD, can last for months to years, so prophylactic and monitoring procedures must be implemented over a long period. Carvalho-Dias et al. analyzed 24 cases of proven and probable invasive aspergillosis among HSCT recipients and reported, that 83% of the patients died due to invasive fungal infection within 60 days of follow-up [72].

Kojima et al. compared the incidence of IA and mortality rates due to this disease in 664 recipients of alloHSCT—486 conventional stem cell transplantation (CST) patients and 178 reduced-intensity stem cell transplant (RIST) recipients. The overall incidence of IA in all 664 recipients of alloHSCT was 35 (5.3%) [74]. Despite significant differences in the estimated 3-year incidence of IA in CST group (4.5%) and RIST population (8.2%) ($P = 0.045$), the mortality rates were similar in both groups (76 and 86%, respectively). However, the median onset of IA after RIST was day 127, which was significantly later than that after CST—day 97 [74]. Furthermore, a multivariate analysis showed that IA was associated with age > 50 years and the presence of acute or chronic GVHD [74]. In another study, Labbe et al. analyzed the risk factors for IA in 125 alloHSCT recipients with nonmyeloablative (NMA) regimens, who received a 6/6 matched sibling NMA HSCT and were treated homogenously [73]. IA developed in 13 patients (5 proved, 6 probable, and 2 possible IA), at 44–791 days (median 229 days) after NMA HSCT. The risk of IA was calculated as 7% at 1 year, 11% at 2 years, and 15% at 3 years after NMA alloHSCT [73]. It was concluded that in NMA HSCT recipients the risk of IA increases over time and is significantly associated with intestinal GVHD, therefore these patients should be monitored for this complication and administration of antifungal prophylaxis with activity against molds should be considered [73].

4.2 Lung and heart-lung transplant recipients

In lung transplant recipients, invasive aspergillosis is the predominant fungal infection [44, 71, 75]. In the past, the incidence of IA in this group of patients was reported in the range of 4.0–23.3%, however, newer studies point to a lower frequency of this disease [44]. On the other hand, the time from lung transplantation to the onset of IA becomes longer due to the use of antifungal prophylaxis in the early post-transplant period. Therefore the median time to IA onset has increased from 120 days post-transplant to 483 or 508 days post-transplant reported in recent studies [44].

The most common species linked to the etiology of IA in lung transplant recipients is *Aspergillus fumigatus*. In an international, multicenter, retrospective cohort study of 900 consecutive adult lung transplant recipients with 4 years of follow-up, 79 patients developed 115 episodes of IA [75]. *Aspergillus fumigatus* was isolated in 72 of 115 (63%) episodes [75]. In a retrospective study of 251 lung transplant recipients, *Aspergillus* was isolated from 86 (33%) cases including 50 patients colonized with *Aspergillus* spp., 17 recipients with tracheobronchitis, and 19 cases of IA [76]. These authors reported that isolation of *Aspergillus* spp. from respiratory samples preceded acute rejection of the graft, therefore it may be a marker of threatening graft rejection and/or inflammation of the airways [76].

The significance of the patient's airway colonization with *Aspergillus* spp. before lung transplantation remains controversial. Some authors indicate its importance within the first year after lung transplantation, if the recipient was colonized in the period of 6 months before lung transplantation, while others did not find any significant link between *Aspergillus* pre-transplant colonization and occurrence of IA in the post-transplant period [44, 75–77]. Other risk factors for IA, which are unique to lung transplant recipients, comprise bronchial anastomotic leaks and other complications within the surgical site, airway narrowing, allograft dysfunction and/or graft ischaemia, reperfusion injury, CMV infection, bronchiolitis, and requirement for more intensive immunosuppressive therapy to prevent graft rejection [44, 76]. In lung transplant recipients, recovery of *Aspergillus* spp. from a respiratory tract sample warrants bronchoscopy to exclude the presence of tracheobronchitis [44].

It should be beared in mind that in lung transplant recipients there is a continuous exposure of the graft to the external environment through the airways, with impaired defense mechanisms (decreased mucociliary function, weakened cough reflex) in the early postransplant period [44].

In lung transplant recipients, there is a transient devascularization of the bronchial anastomotic site, which may contribute to ischemic injury and necrosis. This is a risk factor for development of ulcerative tracheobronchitis—a locally invasive form of IA involving the anastomotic site, the trachea, and the bronchi [44, 78]. In these patients, bronchovascular fistulas may develop, with a potentially fatal hemorrhage.

In the literature reports, the mortality rate of lung transplant recipients with IA ranges from 23 to 29% in individuals with tracheobronchitis to as high as 67–82% in patients with invasive pulmonary aspergillosis, but according to some estimates at present, it could be as low as 20% [44]. In a follow-up study of 251 lung transplant recipients, *Aspergillus* infection was associated with a reduced 5-year survival rate of these patients [76]. Prognosis is worse in patients with aspergillosis of the central nervous system or with disseminated disease [71].

4.3 Heart transplant recipients

According to the literature, the incidence of invasive aspergillosis in heart transplant recipients ranges from 1 to 14% [44, 79]. In this population, the risk factors for IA comprise isolation of *Aspergillus fumigatus* from bronchoalveolar lavage fluid, disease caused by cytomegalovirus, reoperation, and post-transplant hemodialysis [44]. The mortality rate in heart transplant recipients with invasive aspergillosis remains high—in the range of 66–88% [44, 79–81].

Invasive pulmonary aspergillosis remains the most common clinical presentation of this disease, particularly in early-onset IA (≤3 months after transplantation), while in late-onset IA, there is a higher frequency of disseminated disease and involvement of the central nervous system and other extrapulmonary sites [79, 80]. In an analysis of 455 heart transplant recipients, in whom 8 cases of IA have been diagnosed, all had invasive pulmonary form of the disease [79]. Risk factors for early-onset IA (within ≤3 months after heart transplantation), comprised hemodialysis, thoracic reoperation, and the presence of another case in the institution within the preceding 3 months [79]. For late-onset IA in this population of heart transplant recipients, hemodialysis and augmented immunosuppression were identified as risk factors [79]. In the clinical course of these cases, predominated septic shock and multiple organ dysfunction syndrome (MODS), nonspecific clinical and radiographic findings, as well as rapid (at a median of 11 days after diagnosis) mortality despite administration of antifungal therapy with activity against molds [79]. In a study by Montoya et al., none of the heart transplant recipients with either invasive pulmonary aspergillosis or invasive extrapulmonary aspergillosis had neutropenia [81]. Therefore, even in the absence of neutropenia invasive pulmonary aspergillosis should be suspected, particularly within the first 3 months of transplantation in heart transplant recipients who have fever and respiratory symptoms, a positive result of culture of respiratory secretions, and abnormal radiological findings (particularly nodules) [81].

A study of 479 consecutive heart transplant recipients in a single institution revealed a decrease in the incidence of IA from 8.7% (24/277) in the period 1988–2000 to 3.5% (7/202) in 2001–2011 [80]. Overall the incidence of IA in the studied group of heart transplant recipients was 6.5% (31 of 479). However, the authors report that four of seven cases were diagnosed as an outbreak, which indicates that favorable conditions for an infection with *Aspergillus* spp. may be present in a hospital [80]. Over the study period, there was a decrease in the mortality rate among the heart transplant recipients with IA from 46 to 0% ($p = 0.04$) [80]. The authors also noted a higher mortality rate in late-onset IA cases (63%) in comparison to early-onset IA (26%, $p = 0.09$) [80].

4.4 Liver transplant recipients

Invasive aspergillosis is reported in 1.0–9.2% of the liver transplant recipients. Mortality rates have decreased from 83–88% in earlier studies to 33–65% in more recent reports [44]. However, they remain very high in patients who develop invasive aspergillosis after liver retransplantation (82.4%), particularly in those undergoing surgery later than 30 days after primary liver transplantation (100%) [44].

Risk factors for invasive fungal infections, including aspergillosis, in these patients, comprise retransplantation (30-fold higher risk) and renal dysfunction, particularly requiring any form of renal replacement therapy (15- to 25-fold higher risk) [44]. Furthermore, transplantation for fulminant hepatic failure, pretransplant corticosteroid therapy, cytomegalovirus (CMV) infection, and prolonged intensive unit care stay are other risk factors associated with invasive aspergillosis in liver transplant recipients [44]. It is underlined that liver transplant recipients are particularly susceptible to disseminated and central nervous system invasive aspergillosis [44].

Previously most invasive fungal infections in liver transplant recipients occurred within the first month after transplantation (the median time to onset was reported as 16–17 days), however, in recent years, they are usually diagnosed in the late period (>90 days) after liver transplantation. After renal replacement therapy and retransplantation, the median time to onset of IA was reported as 13 and 28 days, respectively [44].

4.5 Kidney transplant recipients

Invasive aspergillosis has been reported in 0.7–4.0% of the renal transplant recipients [44]. It should be emphasized that despite a relatively low overall incidence of IA in comparison to other solid organ transplant (SOT) recipients, the mortality rate is high in these patients—in the range of 67–75% [44]. Risk factors for invasive aspergillosis in kidney transplant recipients are the following: potent immunosuppressive therapy, leukopenia, prolonged and/or high dose corticosteroid therapy, longer duration of renal replacement therapy in the pretransplant period, and graft failure requiring hemodialysis [44, 82].

In a recent study, Desbois et al. analyzed the outcome of IA in kidney transplant recipients in the era of voriconazole availability [83]. Unfortunately, they concluded that the prognosis of patients with IA after renal transplantation is still poor, and even if the patients survive, the risk of graft loss is high [83].

5. Mycological diagnostics

The diagnosis of invasive aspergillosis remains a significant challenge [19]. It is usually based on a histopathological evidence of tissue invasion, in conjunction with an isolation of *Aspergillus* spp. in culture of the biopsy material or other clinically relevant specimen, as well as compatible clinical signs and symptoms in a patient with recognized risk factors. Imaging examinations (radiographic, computed tomography, and magnetic resonance), as well as serological tests (detection of fungal antigens and antifungal antibodies), provide only additional information and should be interpreted in conjunction with the clinical picture and the results of additional laboratory tests [13, 19, 48].

It should be emphasized that fast detection and identification of the etiological agent of infection is of utmost importance as it allows an early start of an effective antimicrobial therapy, which improves the patient's chances to survive.

In mycological diagnostics, the culture of the fungus from the site of infection and *in vitro* susceptibility testing of the isolate remain the "gold" standard. A diagnosis of invasive pulmonary aspergillosis comprises detection of the fungal mycelium with histopathological (with the use of different staining techniques) tests and/or positive culture of the relevant material obtained from the lower respiratory tract [5, 6, 13, 15, 19]. In a patient in whom invasive pulmonary aspergillosis is suspected, it is recommended to culture a sample of bronchoalveolar lavage fluid (BALF), obtained as early as possible during the course of infection [5, 6, 13, 19]. It should be emphasized that the result of sputum culture is not an unequivocal proof of invasive infection of the lung parenchyma, because it may represent only colonization of the respiratory tract by the isolated microorganism. It has been reported that among 66 elderly patients in whom *Aspergillus* spp. was cultured from sputum, only 3 individuals had invasive pulmonary aspergillosis [84]. In another study, no *Aspergillus* spp. was cultured from the sputum of 70% of patients with invasive pulmonary aspergillosis confirmed with other reliable methods [8].

Blood cultures are rarely positive in patients with invasive pulmonary aspergillosis [8, 19, 45]. In patients with pulmonary aspergillosis, *Aspergillus* fungaemia was detected in 10.1% (9/89) of them, at a median of 5 days from the onset of clinical symptoms [19]. The diagnostic role of *Aspergillus* fungaemia in patients with an invasive form of infection is limited because blood cultures become positive (if at all) in the late stage of the disease when a microbiological or clinical diagnosis has already been made [19].

In laboratory diagnostics of this form of aspergillosis, detection of *Aspergillus* spp. antigen—galactomannan (GM)—in BALF or in serum, may be useful; however, it should be remembered that it could represent a false positive result [10, 13, 15, 19, 29]. Detection of another fungal antigen which is a constituent of the fungal cell wall—(1–3)-β-D-glucan (BDG)—is a nonspecific marker of fungal infection, being positive in many fungal infections apart from aspergillosis [13]. Molecular methods (e.g. detection of DNA of the strains classified in the genus *Aspergillus* in blood or BALF using PCR technique) are promising, however at present, they are not routinely available in clinical microbiology laboratories, and interpretation of their results requires further analyses [13, 19, 85]. Research is ongoing on the usefulness of serum interleukin-8 concentration as an auxiliary marker in laboratory diagnostics of invasive pulmonary aspergillosis [86]. Therefore, it should be emphasized that diagnosis of invasive pulmonary aspergillosis requires evaluation of the patient's clinical status in conjunction with the results of various examinations—imaging, histological, and mycological, as well as biochemical markers [1, 8, 13, 15, 86].

Laboratory methods currently used in diagnosis of invasive aspergillosis comprise three groups of techniques: detection of fungal invasion in histopathological examination of tissue sections; direct microscopy and isolation of *Aspergillus* spp. in culture of the clinically relevant samples; and noninvasive methods such as serological detection of antigens or nucleic material of *Aspergillus* spp., or detection of antibodies [19, 87].

5.1 Histopathological examination of tissue sections

Histopathological examination of biopsy or autopsy tissue sections confirms the fungal etiology of invasive infections [1, 5, 6, 13, 15, 19]. Tissue sections are usually stained with hematoxylin and eosin, but other staining techniques are also used in practice (e.g. Gomori-Grocott methenamine silver stain, periodic acid-Schiff stain) [2, 88, 89]. Histopathological tissue sections from a patient with invasive easpergillosis of the heart and lung are shown in Sulik-Tyszka et al. [89].

In tissue sections, *Aspergillus* appears as septate hyphae, with dichotomous branching at 45° angles suggestive of *Aspergillus* spp. [2, 19]. Conidiophores and fruiting bodies are rarely seen, except in areas exposed to air, for example, bronchi [19]. Invasive lesions are characterized by an area of necrosis and non-caseating granulomatous inflammation. A characteristic feature of invasive aspergillosis is trespassing of the the fungus into the blood vessels, with subsequent infarction and tissue necrosis.

5.2 Direct microscopic examination, culture, and identification of *Aspergillus* spp.

Clinical samples for isolation of *Aspergillus* spp. in culture depend on the clinical symptoms and suspected localization of infection. In the diagnosis of invasive pulmonary aspergillosis, a lung biopsy or a sample of BALF is recommended. Other specimens, such as bronchial or endotracheal aspirates, pleural fluid, and also sputum may be cultured as well [5, 6, 19]. Blood cultures can be done, but are usually negative. In fact, any suspicious lesion (e.g. cutaneous or skeletal) should be biopsied and cultured for fungi [19].

The direct microscopic examination allows not only rapid detection of the fungus directly in the specimen, but also its preliminary identification.

A universal solid medium for culturing fungi is Sabouraud agar. When culturing a sample obtained from a site which is primarily nonsterile, Sabouraud agar supplemented with chloramphenicol and gentamicin is used. Czapek-Dox agar and 2% malt extract agar are also used, as well as liquid media [19]. Commercially available media are recommended in order to standardize the culture methods.

Identification of the isolates belonging to the genus *Aspergillus* relies on evaluation of the colony morphology and color (both on the upper and reverse sides of the agar plate), and diffusion of the pigment into the medium (**Figure 1**). Matrix-assisted laser desorption/ionization time-of-flight mass spectrometry (MALDI-TOF-MS) technique may be used in the identification of *Aspergillus* spp. and is a promising tool, particularly for the identification of rare species of *Aspergillus* [90, 91]. This method allows a rapid and reliable identification of the isolate and therefore, an early start of effective antifungal therapy.

Interpretation of the mycological culture results is important and depends on the clinical picture [19]. In a routine microbiology laboratory work, most of the isolates of *Aspergillus fumigatus* do not indicate proven or probable infection. However, cultures positive for *Aspergillus fumigatus*, in the appropriate epidemiological and clinical setting, such as highly immunocompromised transplant recipients, are strongly associated with the presence or risk of IA and therefore should not be disregarded [19]. Also, the isolation of *Aspergillus fumigatus* in hematological patients, even from nonsterile samples, is generally regarded as potentially significant [19]. It has been reported that in heart transplant recipients with suspicion of invasive aspergillosis, a culture positive for *Aspergillus* has a positive predictive value (PPV) of 60–70% [92]. Higher PPV (78–91%) was linked to the isolation of *Aspergillus fumigatus*, with a further increase to 88–100% when *Aspergillus fumigatus* is recovered from a respiratory specimen other than sputum [92].

It should be emphasized that in transplant recipient's fungal cultures may be negative, despite disseminated infection, and in invasive aspergillosis, blood cultures are usually negative, even in patients with *Aspergillus* endocarditis [19].

5.3 Serological testing in the diagnosis of aspergillosis

Serological tests are widely used in the laboratory diagnostics of aspergillosis. Conventional methods, such as culture of clinical samples and direct microscopy of the specimens, have low sensitivity and may give positive results in the late stages of the disease [19]. Furthermore, suitable specimens for these methods may be difficult to obtain in severely ill, immunocompromised patients. In recent years,

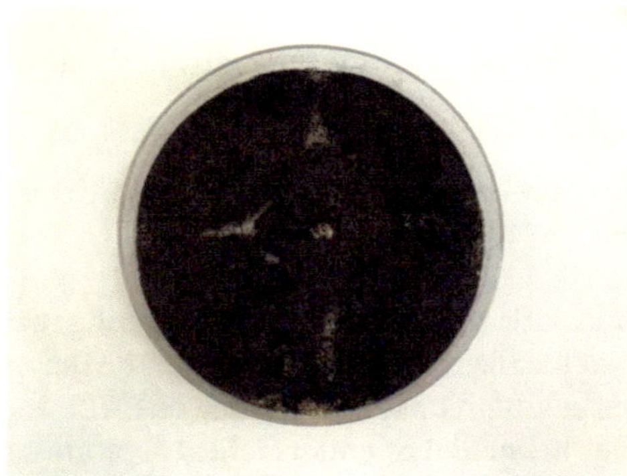

A

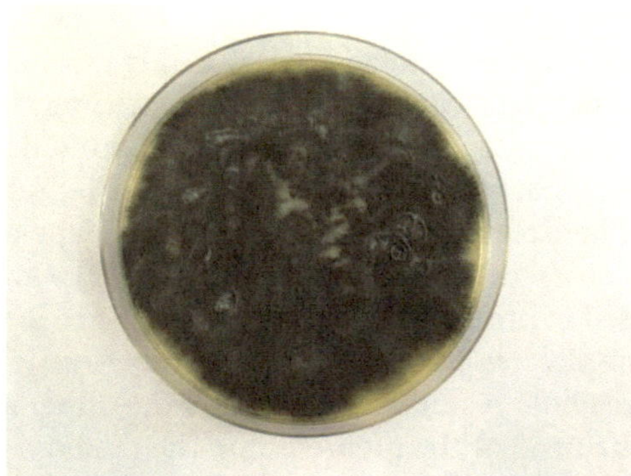

B

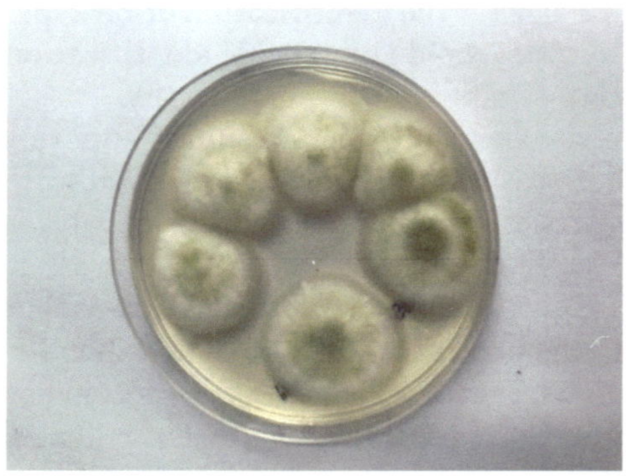

C

Figure 1.
Aspergillus *spp. growth on Sabouraud agar. (A) Aspergillus niger; (B) Aspergillus fumigatus; (C) Aspergillus flavus.*

serological techniques are being used increasingly on such specimens, like serum or BALF, for detection of fungal antigens (e.g. galactomannan, (1,3)-ß-d-glucan) and anti-galactomannan antibodies against *Aspergilllus* [44]. Detection of galactomannan in BALF or serum is at present recommended in the American and European guidelines on laboratory diagnosis of invasive aspergillosis in immunocompromised patients [5, 6, 13].

Duration of antifungal therapy may be guided not only by monitoring of galactomannan levels, but also by the clinical status of the patient and radiological findings.

5.3.1 Galactomannan (GM)

Galactomannan (GM) is a cell wall component of *Aspergillus* spp., released from *Aspergillus* hyphae, while they invade the host tissue, and therefore, it is a specific marker of this fungus [19]. This test may be helpful in early diagnosis of IA (median of 6 days before the symptoms appear) before the infection becomes disseminated [19]. Galactomannan can be detected with the use of latex tests (detection level 15 ng/ml) or more sensitive immunoenzymatic assays, in which 1 ng/ml of GM can be detected. Variation in sensitivity of these tests is being reported, which may due to the different cut-off values for a positive GM result in Europe (1.5 ng/mL) and the USA (0.5 ng/mL) [19].

Galactomannan concentration in the bronchoalveolar lavage fluid, in combination with other diagnostic tests (e.g. chest CT scan or mycological culture) is recommended as a test for the diagnosis of IA in lung and nonlung transplant recipients [71]. Galactomannan in BALF sample has proven superior to serum testing with high sensitivity (67–100%) and specificity rates (91–100%) for the diagnosis of invasive aspergillosis in lung transplant recipients [44]. In patients with prolonged neutropenia and allogeneic stem cell transplant recipients during the early engraftment phase, GM detection is commonly used, and serial screening for GM in serum has a high sensitivity and a negative predictive value for IA [13, 14]. However, serial screening for GM is not recommended in patients receiving antifungal prophylaxis with anti-*Aspergillus* spectrum of activity [13].

False-positive results of galactomannan detection have been documented in up to 13–29% of the liver transplant recipients and in 20% of the lung transplant recipients [44]. In the liver transplant recipients, false-positive results of galactomannan tests were more often seen in patients with transplantation for autoimmune liver disease, perioperative prophylaxis with β-lactam antibiotics, and requirement of dialysis. Most false-positive tests after lung transplantation occurred in the early post-transplant period: that is, in 43% within 3 days, in 64% within 7 days, and in 79% within 14 days of surgery. False-positive results of galactomannan detection are linked to several factors, such as antibiotic therapy with specific groups of antibacterials (such as some cephalosporins, carbapenems, amoxicillin-clavulanate, ampicillin/sulbactam, and piperacillin/tazobactam), cyclophosphamide therapy, as well as administration of blood products, albumin or immunoglobulins, or the use of cellulose hemodialysis membranes [93, 94].

5.3.2 (1,3)-ß-d-glucan

Detection of (1,3)-ß-d-glucan is a nonspecific test for fungal infection, as it is one of the main cell wall polysaccharide components of many fungi [19]. Available diagnostic tests are characterized by a high sensitivity and specificity and enable detection of (1,3)-ß-d-glucan at the concentration of >1 pg/ml. It has been reported that in living-donor, liver allograft recipients, detection of (1,3)-ß-d-glucan was useful for the diagnosis of invasive aspergillosis [95]. Several factors have been linked to false-positive results of the tests for (1,3)-ß-d-glucan, which are similar to those for galactomannan detection [19].

5.4 Molecular methods

At present, molecular diagnostic tests for *Aspergillus* spp. are not available in routine clinical microbiology laboratories, however, in the near future, they will be used increasingly, particularly for identification of unusual species, with specific profiles of susceptibility or resistance to antifungals [19, 44, 96]. Recently, PCR technique for detection of *Aspergillus* spp. has been extensively validated and will be included in the diagnostic criteria in the revised European Organization for Research and Treatment of Cancer/Mycoses Study Group (EORTC-MSG) definitions [97]. A comprehensive review of the molecular diagnosis of invasive aspergillosis has recently been published [85].

The majority of molecular methods which can be used in the clinical microbiology laboratories are based on PCR technique. These methods are particularly useful for testing of lung specimens. It has been reported, that quantitative PCR test used for diagnosis of IA with a sample of bronchoalveolar lavage fluid was characterized by 67% sensitivity and 100% specificity [98]. Perhaps in the future, quantitative PCR tests will also be used to monitor the response to antifungal treatment in patients with IA [19].

Fluorescence in situ hybridization-based molecular method is a promising approach in the *A. fumigatus* detection in the tissues [87]. Species identification of *Aspergillus* isolates may be made by β-tubulin and calmodulin gene sequencing [91]. Further analyses are needed to evaluate the significance of the results of molecular tests in immunocompromised patients suspected of invasive aspergillosis.

6. Treatment of invasive aspergillosis

Successful treatment of invasive aspergillosis comprises early diagnosis of the disease, selection of an appropriate antifungal agent active against fungi of the genus *Aspergillus*, and prompt initiation of antifungal therapy, as well as surgical debridement, particularly in immunocompromised patients, such as HSCT and SOT recipients [3, 44]. Proper pharmacokinetics, pharmacoeconomics, and no interactions with other medications (e.g. immunosuppressants) administered to the patient are further factors which determine the choice of a proper antifungal agent.

At present, there are three groups of antifungal agents, which can be used in the therapy of aspergillosis: azoles, polyenes, and echinocandins [99]. The choice of treatment regimen depends on several factors, including the host's immune status, liver, and kidney functions, and prior antifungal therapies [99]. Treatment regimens of invasive aspergillosis are shown in **Figure 2**.

It should be emphasized that in the choice of proper antifungal therapy, susceptibility testing of the cultured isolate is important in view of an emerging resistance of some *Aspergillus* strains to azoles, as well as identification to the species level, as resistance to antifungals is more likely with certain species of *Aspergillus* other than *Aspergillus fumigatus* [99]. For example, *A. terreus* has a high minimum inhibitory concentration (MIC) to amphotericin B, while *A. calidoustus* has to numerous antifungals [99]. The role of a combination antifungal treatment for primary therapy of IA remains controversial; however, it may be considered (e.g. voriconazole with an echinocandin) for treatment of infection caused by these species [71, 99].

Apart from antifungal therapy, surgery may be indicated in patients with invasive aspergillosis. It applies to the cases in which the disease is localized and infection site is easily accessible to debridement (e.g. invasive fungal sinusitis or localized cutaneous lesions) [5, 6]. Surgical excision or debridement may be used for both diagnostic and therapeutic purposes [44].

Surgery of the sinuses may involve removal of the granulation tissue and necrotic bone [3]. Surgery may also be required in patients with endocarditis, osteomyelitis, or focal lesions in the central nervous system [5, 6]. Surgery is particularly indicated for persistent, or a life-threatening hemoptysis, lesions in the proximity

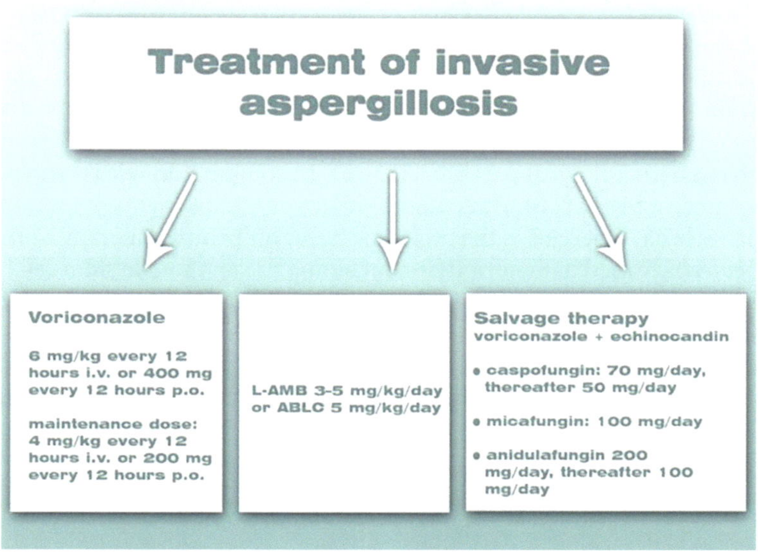

Figure 2.
Treatment of invasive aspergillosis.

of great vessels or pericardium, nasal and sinus infections, single cavitary lesion in the lung, intracranial abscesses, as well as lesions invading the pericardium, bone, the subcutaneous, or thoracic tissue [100].

6.1 Triazoles

According to the newest guidelines of ECIL-6 (the European Conference on Infections in Leukemia), recommendations of Infectious Diseases Society of America (IDSA) and European Society of Clinical Microbiology and Infectious Diseases, European Confederation of Medical Mycology, European Respiratory Society (ESCMID/ECMM/ERS) as well as expert groups, the drugs of first choice in therapy of invasive aspergillosis are triazoles—voriconazole or isavuconazole in monotherapy [5, 6, 13, 20, 71].

Isavuconazole is as effective as voriconazole, and in addition, it is characterized by a better safety profile, therefore in the newest guidelines, it has been granted AI recommendation equally with voriconazole [5, 6]. In patients who do not tolerate voriconazole, therapy with itraconazole or posaconazole may be considered; however, cross-resistance between azoles may be a problem [5]. An alternative antifungal agent used in the therapy of this disease is liposomal amphotericin B [5, 6, 13, 71]. It is emphasized that the chosen agent should be implemented as quickly as possible after fungal etiology of the infection has been suspected [5, 15]. At present, the routine use of combination therapy is neither recommended as a first line treatment, nor the use of echinocandins as the primary treatment [5].

In recent years, an increase in the percentage of strains of *Aspergillus fumigatus* resistant to azoles (including voriconazole) is being observed, which may pose a therapeutic problem [20, 101–103]. Resistance is mainly due to mutations in the gene *cyp51A* and/or overexpression of the efflux pumps in the cells of these fungi [101–106]. Lestrade et al. showed that among 196 patients with IA, in 37 (19%) infection was caused by a strain of *A. fumigatus* resistant to voriconazole, which was linked to >20% increase in the mortality rate in this group of patients in comparison to individuals who received proper antifungal treatment [107]. In 2006–2016, Borman et al. analyzed 2501 clinical strains of *Aspergillus fumigatus*, among which

3.1% were resistant to voriconazole and 12.5% were resistant to amphotericin B [108]. The range of MIC values for these strains to voriconazole was 0.03–16.0 μg/ml and to amphotericin B was 0.06–4.0 μg/ml [108]. In a study comprising 105 clinical strains of *Aspergillus fumigatus*, a significant difference was reported in the percentage of strains resistant to triazoles among the isolates cultured from samples obtained from hematological patients (15.9%), in comparison with the group of patients treated in the ICU (4.5% strains) [101].

Voriconazole has emerged as the preferred agent for primary therapy of IA. Its efficacy has been confirmed in many studies, including hematopoietic stem cell transplant recipients and patients with hematological malignancies, as well as SOT recipients [44]. Voriconazole was effective in heart transplant recipients, in SOT recipients with central nervous system aspergillosis. In a lung transplant patient with *Aspergillus* endophthalmitis, voriconazole has been used in the form of an intravitreal injection [44].

6.2 Liposomal amphotericin B

An alternative antifungal agent recommended in therapy of IA is liposomal amphotericin B (L-AmB), which is active *in vitro* against the majority of strains of *Aspergillus* [5, 6, 13, 44, 71, 99]. However, it should be remembered that some species of *Aspergillus* (e.g. A. *terreus*) neutropaenic patients may be resistant to this antifungal agent.

6.3 Echinocandins

Echinocandins (caspofungin, micafungin, or anidulafungin) are not recommended as first-line therapy of invasive aspergillosis, as they exhibit only fungistatic (not fungicidal) activity against the isolates of *Aspergillus* spp. They can be considered in salvage therapy; however, in combination with voriconazole, isavuconazole, or liposomal amphotericin B [44, 99, 109].

6.4 Salvage therapy

In patients not responding to monotherapy with antifungal agents recommended as first-line therapy, such as voriconazole, isavuconazole, or liposomal amphotericin B, a salvage therapy must be considered, with the use of a combination antifungal regimen [99]. In these cases, it is suggested to combine an echinocandin (caspofungin, micafungin, or anidulafungin) with voriconazole, isavuconazole, or liposomal amphotericin B, while there are no clinical data to support the use of triazoles in combination with amphotericin B [99]. Apart from salvage antifungal therapy, reduction of the doses of immunosuppressive agents (if feasible), as well as surgery should be considered in these patients.

6.5 Duration of antifungal therapy

The duration of therapy for IA is usually 12 weeks, but may range from 3 to >50 weeks or may be even lifelong [5, 6, 13, 44]. Many factors may influence it, such as the response to administered therapy, the patient's immune status and underlying diseases [44]. It is recommended to continue therapy until all clinical and radiographic abnormalities have resolved, and cultures are negative for *Aspergillus*. In transplant recipients, it is important to lower the doses of immunosuppressive agents, as well as to monitor an allograft function [44]. Patterson et al. and other expert groups recommend that therapy of invasive pulmonary aspergillosis should be continued for at least 6–12 weeks, depending on the site of disease, degree and duration of immunosuppression, and evidence of improvement of the patient's clinical status [5, 6]. In patients with stable and pharmacokinetically predictable status, physicians should consider switching from intravenous to oral therapy [13]. If immunosuppression has to be continued after successful therapy of invasive aspergillosis, secondary prophylaxis should be initiated to prevent recurrence of the infection [5, 6].

6.6 Prophylaxis of invasive aspergillosis in transplant recipients

Antifungal prophylaxis against aspergillosis should be used in patients at high risk of IA during prolonged neutropenia [5, 6]. It is recommended to administer posaconazole, voriconazole, or micafungin (caspofungin is also probably effective) [5, 6]. Prophylaxis with itraconazole is effective, but absorption and tolerability of this drug may be a problem.

For allogeneic HSCT recipients with graft-versus-host disease (GVHD), who are at high risk for IA, prophylaxis with posaconazole is recommended, but other azoles active against *Aspergillus* may also be used [5, 6]. In patients with chronic immunosuppression associated with GVHD antifungal prophylaxis should be continued throughout the duration of immunosuppression [5, 6].

According to the ECIL-6 and other recommendations, antifungal prophylaxis with either a systemic triazole (voriconazole or itraconazole) or an inhaled AmB product is recommended for 3–4 months after lung transplantation [5, 6]. Aerosolized amphotericin B is an option which allows the direct administration of the antifungal agent into the transplanted lung, with avoidance of systemic unwanted effects and drug–drug interactions [44]. However, for certain groups of lung transplant recipients (single lung transplant recipients, mold colonization before or after lung transplantation, mold infections detected in explanted lungs, and fungal infections of the sinus) systemic voriconazole or itraconazole is recommended rather than inhaled AmB. Patterson et al. and other experts recommend reinitiation of antifungal prophylaxis in lung transplant recipients who receive immunosuppression augmentation with thymoglobulin, alemtuzumab, or high-dose corticosteroids [5, 6].

For other SOT recipients, antifungal prophylaxis against IA is not routinely recommended and should be based on the institutional epidemiology of aspergillosis and assessment of the patient's risk factors [5, 6, 44]. A common approach to antifungal prophylaxis in liver transplant recipients is to target high-risk patients (fulminant hepatic failure, reoperation, retransplantation, or with renal failure), and it is administered during pre-transplant hospitalization and for the first-month posttransplant. Risk factors for IA have also been identified in heart transplant recipients, such as pretransplant colonization with *Aspergillus* spp., reoperation, cytomegalovirus (CMV) infection, and renal dysfunction. Other risk factors for IA, which may justify antifungal prophylaxis are institutional outbreaks and prolonged or high-dose corticosteroid therapy; however, the optimal duration of such prophylaxis has not been determined [5, 6].

6.7 Immunomodulatory agents and new therapeutic options

At present, it is recommended to reduce the doses of immunosuppressive therapy administered to the patient (or eliminate it, if possible), as this improves the outcome of anti-*Aspergillus* therapy [5, 6]. Other approaches can be considered in cases not responding to standard antifungal therapy, such as granulocyte transfusions in neutropenic patients with IA, or recombinant interferon-γ as prophylaxis in patients with chronic granulomatous disease (CGD) [5, 6].

A relatively new approach to the therapy of invasive aspergillosis in immunocompromised patients involves the use of immunomodulatory agents which would enhance the host's immune system [44]. There is a potential for clinical use of selected cytokines or colony-stimulating factors (e.g. granulocyte colony-stimulating factor, G-CSF; granulocyte-macrophage colony-stimulating factor, GM-CSF; interferon-γ) with immunomodulatory effect [44, 110].

There is an ongoing search for new, more effective antifungals, which will be active also against drug-resistant isolates of *Aspergillus* spp. Currently, there are new classes of antifungal drugs under development—two agents in phase 2 study for the therapy of systemic invasive fungal infections and one drug in phase 1 [111]. Among them are agents which show activity against resistant to azoles *cyp51A* mutants of *Aspergillus* spp.

7. Summary

Diagnosis of invasive aspergillosis remains a challenge for clinicians and microbiologists. Progress in modern diagnostic methods and imaging techniques may contribute to an early and reliable diagnosis of infections caused by *Aspergillus* spp. This is particularly important in immunocompromised patients, such as HSCT and SOT recipients. Proper choice and early commencement of antifungal therapy increase the chances for survival and recovery of these patients from invasive aspergillosis.

Author details

Marta Wróblewska[1,2*], Beata Sulik-Tyszka[1,2], Wojciech Figiel[3], Grzegorz Niewiński[4,5] and Krzysztof Zieniewicz[3]

1 Department of Dental Microbiology, Medical University of Warsaw, Warsaw, Poland

2 Department of Microbiology, Central Clinical Hospital, University Clinical Centre, Medical University of Warsaw, Warsaw, Poland

3 Department of General, Transplantation and Liver Surgery, Medical University of Warsaw, Warsaw, Poland

4 II Department of Anaesthesiology and Intensive Care, Medical University of Warsaw, Warsaw, Poland

5 Intensive Care Unit, Central Clinical Hospital, University Clinical Centre, Medical University of Warsaw, Warsaw, Poland

*Address all correspondence to: marta.wroblewska@wum.edu.pl

References

[1] Davies S, Guidry C, Politano A, Rosenberger L, McLeod M, Hranjec T, et al. *Aspergillus* infections in transplant and non-transplant surgical patients. Surgical Infections. 2014;**15**(3):207-212

[2] Deepa AG, Nair BJ, Sivakumar TT, Joseph AP. Uncommon opportunistic fungal infections of oral cavity: A review. The Journal of Oral and Maxillofacial Pathology. 2014;**18**(2):235-243

[3] Peral-Cagigal B, Redondo-González L-M, Verrier-Hernández A. Invasive maxillary sinus aspergillosis: A case report successfully treated with voriconazole and surgical debridement. Journal of Clinical and Experimental Dentistry. 2014;**6**(4):e448-e451

[4] Richardson M, Bowyer P, Sabino R. The human lung and *Aspergillus*: You are what you breathe in? Medical Mycology. 2019;**57** (Suppl. 2):S145-S154

[5] Patterson TF, Thompson GR, Dening DW, Fishman JA, Hadley S, Herbrecht R, et al. Practice guidelines for the diagnosis and management of aspergillosis: 2016 update by the Infectious Diseases Society of America. Clinical Infectious Diseases. 2016;**63**(4):e1-e60

[6] Tissot F, Agrawal S, Pagano L, Petrikkos G, Groll AH, Skiada A, et al. ECIL-6 guidelines for the treatment of invasive candidiasis, aspergillosis and mucormycosis in leukemia and hematopoietic stem cell transplant patients. Haematologica. 2017;**102**:433-444

[7] Barac A, Ong DSY, Jovancevic L, Peric A, Surda P, Tomic Spiric V, et al. Fungi-induced upper and lower respiratory tract allergic diseases: One entity. Frontiers in Microbiology. 2018;**9**:583

[8] Kousha M, Tadi R, Soubani AO. Pulmonary aspergillosis: A clinical review. European Respiratory Review. 2011;**20**:156-174

[9] Kosmidis C, Denning DW. The clinical spectrum of pulmonary aspergillosis. Thorax. 2015; **70**:270-277

[10] Paramythiotou E, Frantzeskaki F, Flevari A, Armaganidis A, Dimopoulos G. Invasive fungal infections in the ICU: How to approach, how to treat. Molecules. 2014;**19**:1085-1119

[11] Tejerina EE, Abril E, Padilla R. Invasive aspergillosis in critically ill patients: An autopsy study. Mycoses. 2019;**62**(8):673-679

[12] Loreto ES, Tondolo JSM. Epidemiology of Invasive Fungal Infection—An Overview. London, United Kingdom: IntechOpen; 2019. Available from: https://www.intechopen.com/books/fungal-infection

[13] Ullmann AJ, Aguado JM, Arikan-Akdagli S, Denning DW, Groll AH, Lagrou K, et al. Diagnosis and management of *Aspergillus* diseases: Executive summary of the 2017 ESCMID-ECMM-ERS guideline. Clinical Microbiology and Infection. 2018;**24**:e1-e38

[14] Al-Bader N, Sheppard DC. Aspergillosis and stem cell transplantation: An overview of experimental pathogenesis studies. Virulence. 2016;**7**(8):950-966

[15] Jenks JD, Hoenigl M. Treatment of aspergillosis. Journal of Fungi. 2018;**4**(3):98

[16] Cuenca-Estrella M, Kett DH, Wauters J. Defining standards of

CARE for invasive fungal diseases in the ICU. The Journal of Antimicrobial Chemotherapy. 2019;**74**(suppl 2):ii9-ii15

[17] Rudramurthy SM, Paul RA, Chakrabarti A, Mouton JW, Meis JF. Invasive aspergillosis by *Aspergillus flavus*: Epidemiology, diagnosis, antifungal resistance, and management. Journal of Fungi. 2019;**5**(3):55

[18] Lamoth F. *Aspergillus fumigatus*-related species in clinical practice. Frontiers in Microbiology. 2016;7:683

[19] Muñoz P, Guinea J, Bouza E. Update on invasive aspergillosis: Clinical and diagnostic aspects. Clinical Microbiology and Infection. 2006;**12**(suppl. 7):24-39

[20] Lass-Flörl C, Cuenca-Estrella M. Changes in the epidemiological landscape of invasive mould infections and disease. The Journal of Antimicrobial Chemotherapy. 2017;**72**(Suppl 1):i5-i11

[21] Seyedmousavi S, Lionakis MS, Parta M, Peterson SW, Kwon-Chung KJ. Emerging *Aspergillus* species almost exclusively associated with primary immunodeficiencies. Open Forum Infectious Diseases. 2018;**5**(9):ofy213

[22] Sugui JA, Vinh DC, Nardone G, Shea YR, Chang YC, Zelazny AM, et al. *Neosartorya udagawae* (*Aspergillus udagawae*), an emerging agent of aspergillosis: How different is it from *Aspergillus fumigatus*? Journal of Clinical Microbiology. 2010;**48**(1):220-228

[23] van der Linden JWM, Arendrup MC, Warris A, Lagrou K, Pelloux H, Hauser PM, et al. Prospective multicenter international surveillance of azole resistance in *Aspergillus fumigatus*. Emerging Infectious Diseases. 2015;**21**(6):1041-1044

[24] Kalokhe AS, Rouphael N, El Chami MF, Workowski KA, Ganesh G, Jacob JT. *Aspergillus* endocarditis: A review of the literature. International Journal of Infectious Diseases. 2010;**14**(12):e1040-e1047

[25] Kami M, Hori A, Takaue Y, Mutou Y. The gastrointestinal tract is a common target of invasive aspergillosis in patients receiving cytotoxic chemotherapy for hematological malignancy. Clinical Infectious Diseases. 2002;**35**(1):105-106

[26] Shah A, Panjabi C. Allergic bronchopulmonary aspergillosis: A perplexing clinical entity. Allergy, Asthma and Immunology Research. 2016;**8**(4):282-297

[27] Dimopoulos G, Frantzeskaki FG, Poulakou G, Armaganidis AE. Invasive aspergillosis in the intensive care unit. Annals of the New York Academy of Sciences. 2012;**1272**(1):31-39

[28] Bassetti M, Righi E, De Pascale G, De Gaudio R, Giarratano A, Mazzei T, et al. How to manage aspergillosis in non-neutropaenic intensive care unit patients. Critical Care. 2014;**18**:458

[29] Meersseman W, Lagrou K, Maertens J, Wilmer A, Hermans G, Vanderschueren S, et al. Galactomannan in bronchoalveolar lavage fluid: A tool for diagnosing aspergillosis in intensive care unit patients. American Journal of Respiratory and Critical Care Medicine. 2008;**177**:27e34

[30] Nasr WF, Sorour SS, Mobasher MK, Abd El Aziz HR. Chronic sinusitis: A recent histopathological study. International Journal of Otorhinolaryngology Clinics. 2016;**8**(1):1-5

[31] Doloi PK, Baruah DK, Goswami SC, Pathak GK. Primary aspergillosis of the larynx: A case report. Indian Journal of

Otolaryngology and Head and Neck Surgery. 2014;**66**(Suppl 1):326-328

[32] Torul D, Yuceer E, Sumer M, Gun S. Maxillary sinus aspergilloma of odontogenic origin: Report of 2 cases with cone-beam computed tomographic findings and review of the literature. Imaging Science in Dentistry. 2018;**48**(2):139-145

[33] Urs AB, Singh H, Nunia K, Mohanty S, Gupta S. Post endodontic aspergillosis in an immunocompetent individual. Journal of Clinical and Experimental Dentistry. 2015;**7**(4):e535-e539

[34] Sharma D, Mahajan N, Rao S, Khurana N, Jain S. Invasive maxillary aspergillosis masquerading as malignancy in two cases: Utility of cytology as a rapid diagnostic tool. Journal of Cytology. 2012;**29**:194-196

[35] Akhaddar A, Gazzaz M, Albouzidi A, Lmimouni B, Elmostarchid B, Boucetta M. Invasive *Aspergillus terreus* sinusitis with orbitocranial extension: Case report. Surgical Neurology. 2008;**69**:490-495

[36] Arora V, Nagarkar NM, Dass A, Malhotra A. Invasive rhino-orbital aspergillosis. Indian Journal of Otolaryngology and Head and Neck Surgery. 2011;**63**:325-329

[37] Centers for Disease Control and Prevention (CDC). Clinical Features of Aspergillosis. Available from: https://www.cdc.gov/fungal/diseases/aspergillosis/symptoms/clinical-features.html

[38] Wu N, Huang Y, Li Q, Bai C, Huang HD, Yao XP. Isolated invasive *Aspergillus* tracheobronchitis: A clinical study of 19 cases. Clinical Microbiology and Infection. 2010;**16**(6):689-695

[39] Nadkarni T, Goel A. Aspergilloma of the brain: An overview. Journal of Postgraduate Medicine. 2005;**51**:S37-S41

[40] Jantunen E, Salonen J, Juvonen E, Koivunen E, Siitonen T, Lehtinen T, et al. Invasive fungal infections in autologous stem cell transplant recipients: A nation-wide study of 1188 transplanted patients. European Journal of Haematology. 2004;**73**:174-178

[41] Simon DM, Levin S. Infectious complications of solid organ transplantations. Infectious Disease Clinics of North America. 2001;**15**:521-549

[42] Marzolf G, Sabou M, Lannes B, Cotton F, Meyronet D, Galanaud D, et al. Magnetic resonance imaging of cerebral aspergillosis: Imaging and pathological correlations. PLoS One. 2016;**11**(4):e0152475

[43] Singh N, Paterson DL. *Aspergillus* infections in transplant recipients. Clinical Microbiology Reviews. 2005;**18**(1):44-69

[44] Singh NM, Husain S, The AST Infectious Diseases Community of Practice. Aspergillosis in solid organ transplantation. American Journal of Transplantation. 2013;**13**:228-241

[45] Meshaal MS, Labib D, Said K, Hosny M, Hassan M, Abd Al Aziz S, et al. *Aspergillus* endocarditis: Diagnostic criteria and predictors of outcome, a retrospective cohort study. PLoS One. 2018;**13**(8):e0201459

[46] Rofaiel R, Turkistani Y, Mccarty D, Hosseini-Moghaddam SM. Fungal mobile mass on echocardiogram: Native mitral valve *Aspergillus fumigatus* endocarditis. BMJ Case Reports. 2016;**2016**:bcr2016217281

[47] Pierrotti LC, Baddour LM. Fungal endocarditis, 1995-2000. Chest. 2002;**122**:302-310

[48] Paterson DL, Dominguez EA, Chang FY, Snydman DR, Singh N. Infective endocarditis in solid organ transplant recipients. Clinical Infectious Diseases. 1998;**26**:689-694

[49] Woods GL, Wood RP, Shaw BW Jr. *Aspergillus* endocarditis in patients without prior cardiovascular surgery: Report of a case in a liver transplant recipient and review. Reviews of Infectious Diseases. 1989;**11**:263-272

[50] Saxena P, Clarke B, Dunning J. *Aspergillus* endocarditis of the mitral valve in a lung-transplant patient. Texas Heart Institute Journal. 2007;**34**(1):95-97

[51] Mandsager K, Tan C, Menon V. *Aspergillus* prosthetic valve endocarditis. European Heart Journal. 2016;**37**(41):3178

[52] Gumbo T, Taege AJ, Mawhorter S, McHenry MC, Lytle BH, Cosgrove DM, et al. *Aspergillus* valve endocarditis in patients without prior cardiac surgery. Medicine (Baltimore). 2000;**79**:261-268

[53] Bullis SS, Krywanczyk A, Hale AJ. Aspergillosis myocarditis in the immunocompromised host. ID Cases. 2019;**17**:e00567

[54] Yano S. Dilated cardiomyopathy may develop in patients with *Aspergillus* infection. Respiratory Medicine CME. 2010;**3**(4):220-222

[55] Biso S, Lekkham R, Climaco A. *Aspergillus* pericarditis with tamponade in a renal transplant patient. Case Reports in Cardiology. 2017;**2017**:7134586

[56] Comez AT, Komur B, Akcali A, Otkun MT.Ocular aspergillosis: Obtaining a specimen is crucial for diagnosis. A report of three cases. Medical Mycology Case Reports. 2012;**1**(1):39-41

[57] Manikandan P, Abdel-hadi A, Singh YRB, Revathi R, Anita R, Banawas S, et al. Fungal keratitis: Epidemiology, rapid detection, and antifungal susceptibilities of *Fusarium* and *Aspergillus* isolates from corneal scrapings. BioMed Research International. 2019;**2019**:6395840

[58] Hosseini H, Saki S, Saki N, Eghtedari M. *Aspergillus* endophthalmitis in orthotopic liver transplantation. Indian Journal of Medical Sciences. 2009;**63**(6):253-256

[59] Gregory ME, Weir CR, Roberts F, Browne BH. *Aspergillus* endophthalmitis following orthotopic heart transplant. Canadian Journal of Ophthalmology. 2009;**44**(5):607-608

[60] de Machado O, Gonçalves R, Fernandes EM, Campos WR, Oréfice F, Curi AL. Bilateral *Aspergillus* endophthalmitis in a patient with chronic lymphocytic leukaemia. The British Journal of Ophthalmology. 2003;**87**:1429-1430

[61] Fadel FA, Salah DM, Bazaraa HM. Localized renal graft aspergillosis in a child after kidney transplantation: Case report and review of literature. Virology and Mycology. 2016;**5**:3

[62] Haq JA, Khan MA, Afroze N, Haq T. Localized primary renal aspergillosis in a diabetic patient following lithotripsy—A case report. BMC Infectious Diseases. 2007;**7**:58

[63] Singal A, Grover C, Pandhi D, Das S, Jain BK. Nosocomial urinary tract aspergilloma in an immunocompetent host: An unusual occurrence. Indian Journal of Dermatology. 2013;**58**(5):408

[64] Paul S, Singh V, Sankhwar S, Garg M. Renal aspergillosis secondary

to renal instrumentation in immunocompetent patient. BMJ Case Reports. 2013;**2013**:bcr2013200306

[65] Rao P. *Aspergillus* infection in urinary tract post-ureteric stenting. Indian Journal of Medical Microbiology. 2015;**33**:316-318

[66] Zhou L, Zhao H, Chen Z, Zhu L. Urinary tract aspergillosis in a patient with chronic kidney disease. BMJ Case Reports. 2017;**2017**:bcr-2017-221638

[67] Natekar A, Basu S, Mondl G, Pujari M. Cervical aspergillosis in a post-menopausal female: A case report. International Journal of Research in Medical Sciences. 2018;**6**(8):2853-2855

[68] Deb P, Srivastava A. *Aspergillus* in a cervico-vaginal smear of an adult postmenopausal female: An unusual case. Journal of Cytology. 2009;**26**(3):123-124

[69] Li B-K, Wang X, Ding Q. A case report of severe *Aspergillus flavus* penile infection. Asian Journal of Andrology. 2009;**11**(5):638-640

[70] Paterson DL, Singh N. Invasive aspergillosis in transplant recipients. Medicine (Baltimore). 1999;**78**:123-138

[71] Husain S, Camargo JF. Invasive aspergillosis in solid-organ transplant recipients: Guidelines from the American Society of Transplantation Infectious Diseases Community of Practice. Clinical Transplantation. 2019;**33**(9):e13544

[72] Carvalho-Dias VM, Sola CB, Cunha CA, Shimakura SE, Pasquini R, Queiroz-Telles F. Invasive aspergillosis in hematopoietic stem cell transplant recipients: A retrospective analysis. The Brazilian Journal of Infectious Diseases. 2008;**12**(5):385-389

[73] Labbé AC, Su SH, Laverdière M, Pépin J, Patiño C, Cohen S, et al. High incidence of invasive aspergillosis associated with intestinal graft-versus-host disease following nonmyeloablative transplantation. Biology of Blood and Marrow Transplantation. 2007;**13**(10):1192-1200

[74] Kojima R, Kami M, Nannya Y, Kusumi E, Sakai M, Tanaka Y, et al. Incidence of invasive aspergillosis after allogeneic hematopoietic stem cell transplantation with a reduced-intensity regimen compared with transplantation with a conventional regimen. Biology of Blood and Marrow Transplantation. 2004;**10**(9):645-652

[75] Aguilar CA, Hamandi B, Fegbeutel C, Silveira FP, Verschuuren EA, Ussetti P, et al. Clinical risk factors for invasive aspergillosis in lung transplant recipients: Results of an international cohort study. The Journal of Heart and Lung Transplantation. 2018;**37**(10):1226-1234

[76] Solé A, Morant P, Salavert M, Pemán J, Morales P, Valencia Lung Transplant Group. Aspergillus infections in lung transplant recipients: Risk factors and outcome. Clinical Microbiology and Infection. 2005;**11**(5):359-365

[77] Gavalda J, Len O, San Juan R, Aguado J, Fortun J, Lumbreras C, et al. Risk factors for invasive aspergillosis in solid-organ transplant recipients: A case-control study. Clinical Infectious Diseases. 2005;**41**:52-59

[78] Krenke R, Grabczak EM. Tracheobronchial manifestations of *Aspergillus* infections. Scientific World Journal. 2011;**11**:2310-2329

[79] Shields RK, Nguyen MH, Shullo MA, Silveira FP, Kwak EJ, Abdel Massih RC, et al. Invasive

aspergillosis among heart transplant recipients is rare but causes rapid death due to septic shock and multiple organ dysfunction syndrome. Scandinavian Journal of Infectious Diseases. 2012;**44**(12):982-986

[80] Muñoz P, Cerón I, Valerio M, Palomo J, Villa A, Eworo A, et al. Invasive aspergillosis among heart transplant recipients: A 24-year perspective. The Journal of Heart and Lung Transplantation. 2014;**33**(3):278-288

[81] Montoya JG, Chaparro SV, Celis D, Cortés JA, Leung AN, Robbins RC, et al. Invasive aspergillosis in the setting of cardiac transplantation. Clinical Infectious Diseases. 2003;**37**(Suppl 3): S281-S292

[82] Heylen L, Maertens J, Naesens M, Van Wijngaerden E, Lagrou K, Bammens B, et al. Invasive aspergillosis after kidney transplant: Case-control study. Clinical Infectious Diseases. 2015;**60**(10):1505-1511

[83] Desbois AC, Poiree S, Snanoudj R, Bougnoux ME, Sberro-Soussan R, Lanternier F, et al. Prognosis of invasive aspergillosis in kidney transplant recipients: A case-control study. Transplantation direct. 2016;**2**(8):e90

[84] Soubani AO, Khanchandani G, Ahmed HP. Clinical significance of lower respiratory tract *Aspergillus* culture in elderly hospitalized patients. European Journal of Clinical Microbiology and Infectious Diseases. 2004;**23**:491-494

[85] Reyes-Montes MD, Duarte-Escalante E, Frías-De-León MG, Martínez-Herrera EO, Acosta-Altamirano G. Molecular Diagnosis of Invasive Aspergillosis. London, United Kingdom: IntechOpen; 2018. Available from: https://www.intechopen.com/online-first/molecular-diagnosis-of-invasive-aspergillosis

[86] Heldt S, Eigl S, Prattes J, Flick H, Rabensteiner J, Prüller F, et al. Levels of interleukin (IL)-6 and IL-8 are elevated in serum and bronchoalveolar lavage fluid of haematological patients with invasive pulmonary aspergillosis. Mycoses. 2017;**60**(12):818-825

[87] Moura S, Cerqueira L, Almeida A. Invasivepulmonaryaspergillosis:Current diagnostic methodologies and a new molecular approach. European Journal of Clinical Microbiology and Infectious Diseases. 2018;**37**(8):1393-1403

[88] Sulik-Tyszka B, Figiel W, Krawczyk M, Wróblewska M.Invasive aspergillosis of the stomach and co-infection with *Candida krusei* in a patient with terminal liver failure: A case report. Transplantation Proceedings. 2016;**48**(9):3149-3152

[89] Sulik-Tyszka B, Kacprzyk P, Mądry K, Ziarkiewicz-Wróblewska B, Jędrzejczak W, Wróblewska M. Aspergillosis of the heart and lung and review of published reports on fungal endocarditis. Mycopathologia. 2016;**181**:583-588

[90] Vidal-Acuña MR, Ruiz-Pérez de Pipaón M, Torres-Sánchez MJ, Aznar J. Identification of clinical isolates of Aspergillus, including cryptic species, by matrix assisted laser desorption ionization time-of-flight mass spectrometry (MALDI-TOF MS). Medical Mycology. 2018;**56**(7):838-846

[91] Masih A, Singh PK, Kathuria S, Agarwal K, Meis JF, Chowdhary A. Identification by molecular methods and matrix-assisted laser desorption ionization-time of flight mass spectrometry and antifungal susceptibility profiles of clinically significant rare *Aspergillus* species in a referral chest hospital in Delhi, India. The Journal of Clinical Microbiology. 2016;**54**(9):2354-2364

[92] Muñoz P, Alcala L, Sanchez Conde M, Palomo J, Yáñez J, Pelaez T, et al. The isolation of *Aspergillus fumigatus* from respiratory tract specimens in heart transplant recipients is highly predictive of invasive aspergillosis. Transplantation. 2003;**75**:326-329

[93] Boonsarngsuk V, Niyompattama A, Teosirimongkol C, Sriwanichrak K. False-positive serum and bronchoalveolar lavage *Aspergillus* galactomannan assays caused by different antibiotics. Scandinavian Journal of Infectious Diseases. 2010;**42**(6-7):461-468

[94] Tran T, Stacy G, Beal SG. Application of the 1,3-b-D-Glucan (Fungitell) assay in the diagnosis of invasive fungal infections. Archives of Pathology and Laboratory Medicine. 2016;**140**:181-185

[95] Kawagishi N, Satoh K, Enomoto Y. Risk factors and impact of beta-D glucan on invasive fungal infection for the living donor liver transplant recipients. The Tohoku Journal of Experimental Medicine. 2006;**209**:207-215

[96] Dannaoui E, Gabriel F, Gaboyard M, Lagardere G, Audebert L, Quesne G, et al. Molecular diagnosis of invasive aspergillosis and detection of azole resistance by a newly commercialized PCR kit. Journal of Clinical Microbiology. 2017;**55**(11):3210-3218

[97] Patterson TF, Donnelly JP. New concepts in diagnostics for invasive mycoses: Non-culture-based methodologies. Journal of Fungi. 2019;**5**:9

[98] Musher B, Fredricks D, Leisenring W, Balajee SA, Smith C, Marr KA. *Aspergillus* galactomannan enzyme immunoassay and quantitative PCR for diagnosis of invasive aspergillosis with bronchoalveolar lavage fluid. Journal of Clinical Microbiology. 2004;**42**:5517-5522

[99] Kauffman CA. Treatment and Prevention of Invasive Aspergillosis. Alphen aan den Rijn, the Netherlands: Wolters Kluwer; 2019. Available from: https://www.uptodate.com/contents/treatment-and-prevention-of-invasive-aspergillosis

[100] Walsh TJ, Anaissie EJ, Denning DW, Herbrecht R, Kontoyiannis DP, Marr KA, et al. Treatment of aspergillosis: Clinical practice guidelines of the Infectious Diseases Society of America. Clinical Infectious Diseases. 2008;**46**:327-360

[101] Fuhren J, Voskuil WS, Boel CH, Haas PJ, Hagen F, Meis JF, et al. High prevalence of azole resistance in *Aspergillus fumigatus* isolates from high-risk patients. The Journal of Antimicrobial Chemotherapy. 2015;**70**(10):2894-2898

[102] Nawrot U, Sulik-Tyszka B, Kurzyk E, Mroczyńska M, Włodarczyk K, Wróblewska M, et al. Relation of the polymorphism of cyp51A sequence and the susceptibility of *Aspergillus fumigatus* isolates to triazoles determined by commercial gradient test (E-test) and by reference methods. Acta Biochimica Polonica. 2017;**64**(4):631-663

[103] Nawrot U, Kurzyk E, Arendrup MC, Mroczynska M, Wlodarczyk K, Sulik-Tyszka B, et al. Detection of polish clinical *Aspergillus fumigatus* isolates resistant to triazoles. Medical Mycology. 2018;**56**(1):121-124

[104] Spiess B, Postina P, Reinwald M, Cornely OA, Hamprecht A, Hoenigl M, et al. Incidence of *Cyp51 A* key mutations in *Aspergillus fumigatus*—A study on primary clinical samples of immunocompromised patients in the period of 1995-2013. PLoS One. 2014;**9**(7):e103113

[105] Howard SJ, Arendrup MC. Acquired antifungal drug resistance in *Aspergillus fumigatus*: Epidemiology and detection. Medical Mycology. 2011;**49**:90-95

[106] Rajendran R, Mowat E, McCulloch E, Lappin DF, Jones B, Lang S, et al. Azole resistance of *Aspergillus fumigatus* biofilms is partly associated with efflux pump activity. Antimicrobial Agents and Chemotherapy. 2011;**55**(5):2092-2097

[107] Lestrade PP, Bentvelsen RG, Schauwvlieghe AFAD, Schalekamp S, van der Velden WJFM, Kuiper EJ, et al. Voriconazole resistance and mortality in invasive aspergillosis: A multicenter retrospective cohort study. Clinical Infectious Diseases. 2019;**68**:1463

[108] Borman AM, Fraser M, Palmer MD, Szekely A, Houldsworth M, Patterson Z, et al. MIC distributions and evaluation of fungicidal activity for amphotericin B, itraconazole, voriconazole, posaconazole and caspofungin and 20 species of pathogenic filamentous fungi determined using the CLSI broth microdilution method. J Fungi. 2017;**3**(2):E27

[109] Panackal AA. Combination antifungal therapy for invasive aspergillosis revisited. Medical Mycology: Open Access. 2016;**2**(2):12

[110] Delsing CE, Gresnigt MS, Leentjens J, Preijers F, Frager FA, Kox M, et al. Interferon-gamma as adjunctive immunotherapy for invasive fungal infections: A case series. BMC Infectious Diseases. 2014;**14**:166

[111] Sanguinetti M, Posteraro B, Beigelman-Aubry C, Lamoth F, Dunet V, Slavin M, et al. Diagnosis and treatment of invasive fungal infections: Looking ahead. The Journal of Antimicrobial Chemotherapy. 2019;**74**(Suppl 2): ii27-ii37